*The Skidmore-Roth
Outline Series:*

PEDIATRIC NURSING
2nd Edition

Ann Froese-Fretz, R.N., M.S., C.P.N.P.
Theresa Eldridge, R.N., M.S.N., C.P.N.P.
Carole Shega, R.N., M.S., C.P.N.P.

Cathleen M. Kiser, RN, BSN
Community Health Nurse
EDIS, Yokota Air Base, Japan

A SKIDMORE-ROTH PUBLICATION

$\mathcal{SR}$
PUBLISHING

Series Editor: Molly Sullivan, B.A.

Copy Editor: Kathryn Head

Cover Design: Barbara Barr, Visual Impact

Typesetting: Jeannine Parker, Affiliated Executive Systems

Froese-Fretz, Ann
Eldridge, Theresa
Shega, Carole

The Skidmore-Roth Outline Series: Pediatric Nursing/Ann Froese-Fretz, Theresa Eldridge, Carole Shega

ISBN 1-56930-067-4

1. Nursing-Handbooks, Manuals

2. Medical-Handbooks, Manuals

SKIDMORE-ROTH PUBLISHING, INC.
400 Inverness Drive South, Suite 260
Englewood, CO 80112
1-800-825-3150
www.skidmore-roth.com

Table of Contents

Preface

Pediatric patients are a special challenge. They are different psychologically and physiologically and present very different pathophysiologies. Children are also in the process of "becoming" physically, emotionally, and socially. This rapid change affects them not only in terms of bodily appearance and function, but also affects the family unit. They are impacted strongly by what occurs in the world around them, family beliefs about child rearing, socioeconomic status, and disease. Everything impacts on the future adult in the child. Any stressor can alter this process of "becoming" and change the outcome — either positively or negatively — for that child. In order to provide care for children and their families, the nurse must have an understanding of not only the physiology, pathophysiology, and treatment, but also the impact of illness and stress on the child and the family.

This book is designed to provide the reader with an outline for pediatric patient care. It covers all aspects including growth and development, physical assessment, physiology and pathophysiology as well as treatments and commonly used medications. It emphasizes the differences between pediatric and adult patients and also addresses psychosocial care and patient/family education. The text, though appropriate for multiple audiences, is targeted toward nursing students and nurses who do not practice acute care pediatrics on a regular basis. It is useful to provide a basis for further study into selected areas of pediatrics and serves as an outline for an overall picture of commonly encountered problems and solutions in pediatric nursing.

We have attempted to provide a reality-based pediatric text that will provide information based on a "need-to-know" basis. It is designed to heighten awareness of the special challenge that children present. It is our hope that this book will enhance the knowledge base necessary for meeting this challenge.

Each developmental stage is characterized by certain distinct behaviors. These are illustrated in the following table.

Stage	*Characteristic Behaviors*
Infancy	* Period between birth and 18 months * Rapid physical and social growth * Exhibit generalized, reflexive responses to stimuli * Little meaningful purposeful direction to behavior due to immature cerebral cortex * Born with a series of reflex actions that are predictive of later neurological functioning * Increasing brain size allows for performance of increasingly complex behaviors * Play serves as a practice time for development. Becomes increasingly complex as the infant grows * Cognitive development/functioning is difficult to measure and it is accepted that infants function by operant conditioning
Early Childhood	* Period from 18 months - 4 years * Physical growth has slowed but the systems are maturing and becoming more efficient * Eating habits reflect independence. Food "jags" very common - may become a control issue * Toilet training occurs during this time and often becomes source of anxiety for many parents * Can walk, run, jump and move up and down stairs * Fine motor skills increase * Imitates behavior well as learning continues * Imagination is very active and magical thinking is common * By age 3, vocabulary contains approximately 1000 words * Independence asserted -"terrible twos" seen during this time. The favorite word is "no"
Middle Childhood	* Kindergarten through 3rd grade * Great social and cognitive change * Learning occurring at a rapid rate * As many changes physiologically as an infant * Cerebral dominance and "handedness" established by 4.5 years * Gross motor ability more refined and evidenced by ability to throw a ball with one hand, ride a bicycle, and roller skate * Eye-hand coordination and fine motor skills increase * Play is cooperative and associative. Increased ability to share and cooperate with peers. Games more complex — leader and follower skills develop. Symbolic play important * Cognitive development occurs rapidly. Learn by observation and imitation Logical thinking and memory increase. Language skills increase * Decrease in egocentric thinking and child more sensitive to others * Self-concept tied to success * Fear bodily harm and injury * Child discovers parents are fallible
Late Childhood	* 8-12 years * Continue to mature biologically and physiologically * Girls have growth spurt at about 10 years and are taller and heavier than boys until early adolescence * Gross motor skills more organized and purposeful * Play remains important. Very competitive * Long-term memory utilized more as child develops a learning style. Use storytelling to relate events * Sense of humor develops * Independence continues to increase * Heavily rely on parents for praise and support

Adolescence

* Longest period of development
* Period of great change and perhaps turmoil
* Both sexes experience a growth spurt. May occur any time between 10 and 18 years
* Epiphyseal plates of long bones close. Governed by sex hormones. Early or late onset of puberty associated with height or mean
* Body proportions more like those of an adult
* Apocrine sweat glands and sebaceous glands become active during this time
* Three types of play:
  a. cooperative play (games, clubs, and dating);
  b. team play (team sports); and,
  c. construction play (hobbies)
* Cognitive development continues. Can engage in abstract thinking
* Search for self-concept continues. Asks what he/she wants to be

1

GROWTH AND DEVELOPMENT

Children were viewed as little more than "small adults" until the late 1800s. They had little relative value in society and were viewed as property. The head of the household had the power of life and death over the children and could determine their fates even into adulthood. Children were expected to behave as adults, and play was viewed as foolish or sinful. Children were workers and began helping out at home at a very early age. Formal schooling was viewed as a luxury and reserved for males only.

Beginning in the late 19th century and continuing today, several theories have attempted to explain the developmental process. Each theorist has studied different aspects of development. Some focused on physical growth and neurological development while others looked at cognitive and "psychosexual" development. Most modern-day practitioners, however, prefer to utilize a combination of the major theories. Information and the central ideas of each of these theorists are presented in the following table.

DEVELOPMENTAL THEORIST AND CENTRAL IDEA				
AGE	*Freud*	*Erikson*	*Piaget*	*Kohlberg*
Birth - 18 mos.	Oral	Basic Trust vs. Mistrust	Sensorimotor	"Amoral"
18 mos.- 3 years	Anal	Autonomy vs. Shame and Doubt	Symbolic (Preoperational)	Stages 1 - 2
3 - 6 years	Oedipal	Initiative vs. Guilt	Intuition (Preoperational)	Stages 1 - 3
6 - 11 years	Latency	Industry vs. Inferiority	Concrete Operational	Stages 2 -5
12 - 17 years	Adolescence (genital)	Identity vs. Role Confusion	Formal Operational	Stages 4 -6
17 - 30 years	Young Adulthood	Intimacy vs. Isolation	Formal Operational	Stages 4 -6
30 - 60 years	Adulthood	Generativity vs. Stagnation	Formal Operational	Stages 4 -6
60 years & over	Old Age	Ego Integration vs. Despair	Formal Operational	Stages 4 - 6

Growth and development occurs in regular, related patterns that reflect physical development and the maturation of neuromuscular function. These are termed cephalocaudal, proximodistal, and differentiation. **Cephalocaudal patterns** are exhibited by development that begins with the head. It develops first and is very large and complex while the lower end is simpler and develops later (fetal brain develops first; the head is relatively large compared to the overall size of the infant; there is eye use before hand use; and control over hands is gained before control over feet). **Proximodistal development** is illustrated by the "near-to-far" or "midline to peripheral" concept (limb buds develop before toes and fingers, shoulder control occurs before hand and whole hand is mastered before finger control). Central nervous system (CNS) development occurs prior to peripheral nervous system development. **Differentiation** is demonstrated by the fact that simple operations/actions develop first and are followed by more complex operations/actions and broad, global behaviors are followed by the more specific and refined patterns (the embryonic development progresses from undifferentiated cell function to highly differentiated, specialized cell function; gross motor function precedes fine motor function).

There is also a definite, predictable sequence in all dimensions of the growth and development process. This allows for the creation of charts with ranges for developmental milestones and growth. **Orderly and continuous sequential patterns** are noted for all children. Each stage of development is affected by the stages preceding it and will influence all future stages (a child learning to walk creeps, crawls, stands, stands alone, and then walks). The theory of **epigenesis** (development results from the growth and differentiation of specialized cells) is also important to the developmental process. New parts and behaviors arise from those already in existence (the nervous system develops from the neural plate, fingers develop from limb buds, and personality facets build on the development of basic trust).

Finally, it must be remembered that growth and development do not occur at the same rate for all children. "There are periods of accelerated growth and periods of decelerated growth in both total body growth and growth of subsystems" (Whaley and Wong, 1988, p. 101). The focus of growth and development changes with different periods during the development of the child. Body proportions change as the child grows.

Each developmental stage is characterized by certain distinct behaviors. These are illustrated in the following table.

STAGE	CHARACTERISTIC BEHAVIORS
Infancy	* Period between birth and 18 months * Rapid physical and social growth * Exhibit generalized, reflexive responses to stimuli * Little meaningful purposeful direction to behavior due to immature cerebral cortex * Born with a series of reflex actions that are predictive of later neurological functioning * Increasing brain size allows for performance of increasingly complex behaviors * Play serves as a practice time for development. Becomes increasingly complex as the infant grows * Cognitive development/functioning is difficult to measure and it is accepted that infants function by operant conditioning
Early Childhood	* Period from 18 months - 4 years * Physical growth has slowed but the systems are maturing and becoming more efficient * Eating habits reflect independence. Food "jags" very common — may become a control issue * Toilet training occurs during this time and often becomes source of anxiety for many parents * Can walk, run, jump and move up and down stairs * Fine motor skills increase * Imitates behavior; learning continues * Imagination is very active and magical thinking is common * By age 3, vocabulary contains approximately 1000 words * Independence asserted — "terrible twos" seen during this time; the favorite word is "no"
Middle Childhood	* Kindergarten through 3rd grade * Great social and cognitive change * Learning occurring at a rapid rate * As many changes physiologically as an infant * Cerebral dominance and "handedness" established by 4.5 years * Gross motor ability more refined and evidenced by ability to throw a ball with one hand, ride a bicycle, and roller skate * Eye-hand coordination and fine motor skills increase * Play is cooperative and associative. Increased ability to share and cooperate with peers. Games more complex — leader and follower skills develop. Symbolic play important * Cognitive development occurs rapidly. Learn by observation and imitation. Logical thinking and memory increase. Language skills increase * Decrease in egocentric thinking and child more sensitive to others * Self-concept tied to success * Fear bodily harm and injury * Child discovers parents are fallible
Late Childhood	* 8-12 years * Continue to mature biologically and physiologically * Girls have growth spurt at about 10 years and are taller and heavier than boys until early adolescence * Gross motor skills more organized and purposeful * Play remains important. Very competitive * Long-term memory utilized more as child develops a learning style. Use storytelling to relate events * Sense of humor develops * Independence continues to increase * Rely heavily on parents for praise and support

STAGE	CHARACTERISTIC BEHAVIORS
Adolescence	* Longest period of development * Period of great change and turmoil * Both sexes experience a growth spurt. May occur any time between 10 and 18 years * Epiphyseal plates of long bones close. Governed by sex hormones * Early or late onset of puberty associated with extremes of short or tall stature, though onset of puberty may be counteracted by genetically determined shortness or tallness. Mean age at onset of puberty usually results in mean height and weight for sex and age * Body proportions more like those of an adult * Apocrine sweat glands and sebaceous glands become active during this time * Three types of play: a. Cooperative play (games, clubs, and dating) b. Team play (team sports) c. Construction play (hobbies) * Cognitive development continues. Can engage in abstract thinking * Search for self-concept continues. Asks what he/she wants to be

Many factors can adversely affect growth and development. The first of these are **genetic factors**. In order to more fully understand how genetic factors interface with growth and development, one must have a basic understanding of embryology. Although the first studies on embryology were done during the golden age of Greece, many "discoveries" have been recent. As embryos develop, 3 distinct phases are apparent. These are cellular multiplication, cellular differentiation, and organ system development. It is also important to remember that all systems arise from 3 primary germ layers. Each system has a critical period during which **any** disruption can adversely affect growth and development. Most system development occurs during the first trimester and coexisting congenital defects most often arise from the same layer. It is not uncommon to see a "grouping" of defects all arising from the same primary germ layer.

GERM LAYER	STRUCTURES ARISING FROM EACH
Mesoderm	* Supporting structure - connective tissue, bones, cartilage, muscle, tendons * Upper portion of urinary system - kidneys and ureters * Reproductive system * Heart and circulatory system * Blood cells
Endoderm	* Linings of GI and respiratory tracts * Tonsils * Parathyroid, thyroid, and thymus glands * Lower urinary tract (bladder and urethra)
Ectoderm	* Nervous system * Skin, hair and nails * Sense organs * Mucous membranes of anus and mouth

Normally, chromosomes exist in pairs (22 pairs of autosomes plus a pair of sex chromosomes). Chromosomal abnormalities include numerical chromosomal abnormalities (monosomy and trisomy) and structural chromosomal abnormalities (translocation and deletion).

Teratogens can have a great impact on developing embryos. A teratogen is defined as any chemical or physical factor that has an adverse effect on a developing embryo or fetus. Exposure to teratogens is inevitable but the amount of damage done, if any, is influenced by the strength of the teratogen, the time during which it is introduced, and its affinity for tissues or specific systems. Many teratogens have predictable consequences. This knowledge of potential fetal damage allows for maternal education on avoidance and prediction of damage should exposure occur.

Physical factors are important to later development. These include genetic mutations (such as cystic fibrosis and sickle cell anemia), diseases that are the result of interaction between genes and the environment (diabetes), and chronic illness or self-care deficits.

Environmental factors such as poor nutrition and environmental hazards and toxins can adversely affect a developing fetus or a growing child. Poor maternal dietary intake often results in intrauterine growth retardation (IUGR) or a small for gestational age (SGA) infant. Many children in the U.S. receive far less than adequate intake of nutrients necessary for physical growth (including brain growth). This adversely affects long-term mental functioning. Environmental hazards such as pollution have been implicated in the development of chronic illness.

Finally, social, cultural, and affective factors must be considered. These include socioeconomic factors, culture, ethnic origin, and religion/religious practices. Health promotion and preventive care are often neglected in lower socioeconomic families. It is difficult to budget for healthcare if it will deprive the family of food or shelter. Insurance is often too expensive for these families. Cultural beliefs about child rearing, health/health promotion, illness, and medical care must be considered when providing care for pediatric patients. These factors determine the type of affection displayed, the expectations of each age and sex, and the way the child is corrected or disciplined. Finally, religion plays an important role in decisions families make when seeking medical care. Some religions have strict guidelines regarding medical care. These include the refusal of blood products and organ transplants by Jehovah's Witnesses and the search for spiritual healing by Christian Scientists.

2

ILLNESS AND HOSPITALIZATION
OF THE PEDIATRIC PATIENT

I. General Concepts

- Illness and hospitalization is a stressful experience for children and their families

- The pediatric population is at high risk for a variety of illnesses and possible hospitalization due to the immaturity of the body systems and frequent new contacts with other children, animals, and the environment

- Children's reaction to the stress of hospitalization is influenced by their developmental age, support systems available, and previous experience with illness and hospitalization

- Growth and development levels are important to consider when interacting with the ill child

- Communication concerning health and illness should be directed toward the parent and child (preschooler and older)

- The family and nurse will play a significant role in maintaining the child's health and optimal functioning level

- Discharge planning is essential for the pediatric population, since they are dependent on their parents for continued care

II. Illness

- Can be either acute or chronic

- May require home, outpatient or inpatient care

- May be viewed by toddlers and preschoolers as a punishment for bad behavior

- May hinder normal growth and development if it removes the child from his normal active environment

- Causes stress for family and child

- May be influenced by family views, cultures, ethnicity, social class, financial ability, home environment, community, nutrition

  - **Nursing Interventions**
    1. Provide anticipatory guidance to all parents to allow for a sense of control when problems arise.

    2. Focus on prevention, detection, education and evaluations, as well as enhancing the child's growth and development during illness.

    3. Strive to maintain the child in a normal home or school environment when disease occurs and attempt to prevent disease progression requiring hospitalization.

III. Hospitalization

Communication

1. **Assess Age and Understanding Level of Child**

2. **Age-Specific Suggestions**
   a. **Infants** — Use nonverbal communication, discuss with parents procedures, illness. Infants are very aware when parents become upset or fearful and will respond accordingly.

   b. **Toddlers and preschoolers** — Very egocentric, need to know what they can do or what will happen to them, let them play with equipment. Give them as much control as possible. They communicate by pulling objects toward them or pushing them away. Use simple and short sentences, describe things completely and realize they understand everything literally, several explanations may be required.

   c. **Schoolage** — Require explanations for everything, communication well-developed but continue to use simple terms, pictures, doll play. Explain what will happen to them, how they can help, and what will happen afterwards.

   d. **Adolescents** — Understand all communication but not necessarily medical terms. Utilize pictures, equipment prior to treatments and procedures, encourage questions. Ensure confidentiality and privacy.

Admission

1. Familiarize child and parent with room, roommate, nurses, and where supplies are stored (diapers, towels, sheets, blankets).

2. Describe hospital routines (change of shifts, times of rounds, mealtimes).

3. Encourage parent and child to do as much for selves and child as is permitted. Give the child as much control over care as possible.

4. Describe all equipment and limitations it poses on child.

5. Inform of safety precautions while in hospital (keeping siderails up, not playing with equipment).

6. Encourage preadmission tours, if possible, to allow for exploring by parent and child in a non-threatening manner.

7. Attempt to staff same nurses to care for child and provide continuity in care.

Medication Administration

1. Explain procedures to parents and child; encourage questions.

2. Pediatric medication doses are ordered as milligrams/kilogram of body weight. All doses should be checked for accuracy prior to administration. This includes comparison of ordered mg/kg to recommended dose.

3. If only adult doses are available, pediatric doses may be calculated by using Clark's Rule:

$$\text{Estimated child's dose} = \frac{\text{weight of child (lbs) x adult dose}}{150 \text{ lbs}}$$

4. PO medication:
    a. Position child according to age.
    b. Administer liquids with oral syringe into side of mouth or cheek, or with nipple for infants; and, by spoon or medicine cup for toddlers and older children.
    c. Because it is difficult for young children to swallow pills, medications should be administered in liquid form (elixir or suspension). These may also be used with older children who are unable to swallow pills or capsules.
    d. If administering with food, consider these guidelines:
        – Will the medication alter the taste of the food?
        – Always use a "nonessential" food such as applesauce

- Mix with only a small amount of food or formula (in case the child takes only a small amount) and feed to the child prior to offering other foods
- Don't give honey to children under 2 years old to avoid the chance of infantile botulism

IM Injections

1. Assess age and size of child, visualize muscle group to be used.

2. Apply the topical anesthetic EMLA to the injection site for a minimum of one hour, preferably up to two hours, prior to injection when possible.

3. Employ assistance to restrain child as needed to prevent unnecessary trauma.

4. Consider the following muscle groups:
   a. Infants and toddlers: vastus lateralis
   b. Preschoolers: vastus lateralis or dorso gluteal
   c. School-age and adolescents: dorso gluteal, deltoid, ventrogluteal

5. Choose the needle length and gauge according to the kind of medication, the amount of medication, and the muscle being injected. The amount of subcutaneous fat, and the viscosity of the medication must be considered.

6. Wear gloves for administration.

7. Explain what child should expect and how long it will take.

8. Complete as quickly as possible.

9. Apply a bandage.

10. Praise the child's attempt to cooperate.

IV Initiation and Maintenance

1. Select site which will be least limiting to patient for age, and which is easily visible for inspection. Sites frequently used include:
   a. Infants: scalp, feet, hands
   b. Toddlers: scalp, non-dominant hand/arm
   c. Preschoolers and older: non-dominant hand or forearm

2. Use non-dominant extremity and allow child to choose site when possible.

3. Apply the topical anesthetic EMLA to the injection site for a minimum of one hour, preferably up to two hours, prior to injection when possible.

4. Explain procedure to child and parent, naming the site, sensations, length of time IV will be in place, and activities child will still be able to do (ambulate, play, shower).

5. Select catheter according to child's size and the viscosity of IV fluid (usually 21-24 gauge is preferred).

6. Prepare all supplies and obtain assistance from other staff with young children who may not be able to cooperate. Allow parents to leave the room if unable to cope with procedure.

7. Secure catheter and tubing (utilize armboards, splints, tape, mitts prn).

8. Monitor site for redness, swelling, induration, or disconnection every hour, provide site care as required by the policy and procedures of the institution.

9. Remember pediatric patients become dehydrated or overhydrated rather quickly, therefore, monitor intake and output, skin status, and lung sounds carefully.

10. Utilize IV pump and Buretrol to allow for closer monitoring of fluid administration and prevention of dehydration or overhydration.

11. Ensure that IV is running according to physician order and within prescribed maintenance rate guidelines:
    * 0 - 10 kg: 100 cc/kg/day
    * >10 - 20 kg: 1000 cc/day for the first 10 kg of body weight plus an additional 50 cc/kg/day for every kg between 10 and 20
    * >20 kg: 1500 cc/day for the first 20 kg of body weight plus an additional 20 cc/kg/day for each kg greater than 20
    ** The hourly rate is obtained by dividing the daily volume by 24 hours.

12. If administering IV medications, alter the IV rate to give the medication only as a last resort (volume or time should be changed first).

IV. Treatments and Procedures

1. Explain all treatments and procedures to parents and child.

2. Allow play and experimentation with equipment when possible.

3. Never ask parents to secure child during painful procedure.

4. Special procedures:
   a. LAB WORK
      – Have all materials assembled
      – Explain purpose and procedure to parent and child

- Secure child and perform procedure as quickly as possible
- Apply adhesive bandage and pressure
- Praise child's attempts to cooperate

b. CATHETERIZATION (URINARY)
  - Often very threatening to parent and child
  - Have all materials assembled
  - Explain procedure to parent and child
  - Provide for privacy
  - Secure child and perform procedure as quickly as possible
  - Secure catheter to child and check placement regularly
  - Perform catheter care as required by the policies and procedures of the institution
  - Praise child's attempts to cooperate

V. Stressors From Hospitalization

1. Reactions According To Age

a. Infants — Infants adapt well if fed, touched, and cared for; in later infancy they experience separation anxiety, exhibit total body rigidity, protest, detach from parents, exhibit withdrawal behavior.

  - **Nursing Interventions:** Encourage parents to stay with, visit, and continue routines of home care for infant as much as possible; establish a sense of trust; maintain same nurse assignments; speak to, look at, and touch infant; provide comfort source as needed (pacifier, bottle, blanket); make environment safe (siderails up, equipment out of reach); attempt to maintain routines; monitor growth and development and provide appropriate interactions and toys.

b. Toddlers — Experience separation anxiety, physically protest and cry, feel a loss of control and rituals, exhibit temper tantrums, exhibit regression, may verbally protest, fear injury and pain, may bite and kick during interaction.

  - **Nursing Interventions**: Encourage parents to stay with, visit, and continue routines of home care as much as possible, establish trust with parents and child, provide familiar routines and items (security objects), maintain same nurse assignment, allow child a sense of independence, allow child to play and interact with family members, stay with child when parents leave so sense of abandonment is not felt, monitor growth and development and provide appropriate interactions and toys (motor development is important during this age).

c. Preschoolers — Experience separation from family but not to the point of anxiety, fear loss of routines and schedules, sense loss of control, fear bodily injury (very active imagination: fantasy, fears and magical thinking), believe all insides can come out any hole in skin (Bandaid® age), exhibit crying, shame, feeling punished, may exhibit regression, aggression, and have nightmares, believe hospitalization is punishment for bad thoughts and actions.

– **Nursing Interventions:** Encourage parents to stay or visit frequently, encourage parents to call child on the phone, provide familiar routines and allow independence in daily care as much as possible, maintain same nurse assignment, allow child to interact and play with others and family, keep night light on during sleep, allow familiar items to be kept with child, explain in simple terms what procedures are going to be done just prior to being done, praise child for accomplishments, utilize play therapy as much as possible to diminish fears, encourage interaction and play with other children in the hospital in age group, monitor growth and development.

d. **Schoolage** — Experience fear of separation from family and friends, getting behind in school, body mutilation, and loss of independence; exhibit stress by attempting to negotiate, crying, fighting, withdrawal, attempting to be brave, ask many questions.

– **Nursing Interventions:** Describe illness, treatments, and procedures to child and parent, encourage family visitation, encourage phone calls, letters, banners from friends and family, allow questions and answer in simple terms, allow independence and choices as much as possible, encourage doing school work, set limits, establish routines, utilize play therapy, tell child crying is O.K., provide child with privacy after procedures to recompose self, encourage rooming with or playing with other children of the same age, monitor growth and development.

e. **Adolescents** — Experience fear of being different, embarrassment, bodily injury, separation from family and friends, loss of privacy, loss of independence, may exhibit overconfidence, withdrawal, noncompliance with regimens, regression, and acting out.

– **Nursing Interventions:** Maintain honest and open communication, provide information regarding illness and treatments, encourage questions and provide understandable answers, provide privacy, encourage interaction with family, friends and others in age group who are hospitalized, assist with maintaining homework, allow decision making as possible, set limits.

Nursing Care for Pediatric Patients

1. **Stressors**

   a. **Altered body image** - Assist with hygiene and care, assess child's self-concept, have child color/draw a picture of self and discuss, ask what would make them feel better and look better and assist with reaching goal.

   b. **Fear of death** — Assess level of understanding and discuss concerns.

Infants — No concept of death, may note separation if loved one dies, unaware that own illness could lead to death.

- **Nursing Interventions:** Support parents, provide information, determine what religious ceremonies are appropriate if infant dies. If infant dies, allow parent to hold child in quiet room, provide a photograph of infant, lock of hair and footprints (if parents do not have these). Utilize infant's name when speaking about infant, actively listen to parents.

Toddlers — No concept of death, may sense separation and impact on routines, may want to visit dead relative, unaware that illness may cause death.

- **Nursing Interventions:** Support parents and child if illness is terminal, provide parents time for questions regarding child's status and give honest answers, provide parents time alone with toddler, utilize toddler's name when speaking of toddler after death, listen.

Preschoolers — Believe death is temporary and reversible, a time of "sleeping"; believe all body functions continue after death; believe illness or death can happen if someone is "bad"; fear how they will go to the bathroom or eat after death; wonder if they will be cold, hungry or be able to play; fear it will hurt to die; may ask if they are going to die due to illness.

- **Nursing Interventions**: Support parent and child if illness is terminal, identify child's beliefs about death and clarify misconceptions utilizing words and terms they can understand, provide comfort and honesty to child and parents, after death allow parent to visit and hold child, ask if there is anything they would like done, actively listen to parents.

Schoolage
6 - 9 years — Personify death (bogeyman), think of death concretely and may wonder if they are going to die when sick, realize body will decay once dead and that death is permanent.
9 - 10 years — Full concept of death develops, may fear own death and see it as unfair, may become aggressive if own death is near, may try to appear strong and unafraid in front of parents, may fear people will see them naked or soil themselves once dead, may ask about what happens after life.

- **Nursing Interventions:** Encourage parent to openly discuss illness and death with child, ask child what death means to them and discuss feelings and fears, encourage parents to allow child as much independence as possible before death, incorporate child in planning of "will" after death and support parents and child's wishes before and after death, allow parent to hold child after death or stay in quiet room, actively listen to parents.

Adolescents — Well-developed concept of death, think it won't happen to them, may still have some magical thinking (death as punishment), may become angry, frustrated, experience denial or become withdrawn when confronted with death.

- **Nursing Interventions:** Support adolescent and parent, give honest, and thorough information, allow adolescent to discuss feelings and wishes or dreams he would like to achieve before death, encourage interaction with other adolescents and friends, allow adolescent to make decisions, as possible; encourage adolescent to assist making plans for after death (what he will wear, flowers), allow parents time with adolescent before and after death, actively listen.

Families of a terminally-ill child — Parents need special support, they often tend to overprotect child and encourage dependency of child on themselves, may isolate selves from spouse, other children or society; need time to talk, ask questions, and go through the grieving process, may abandon the dying child.

- **Nursing Interventions:** Listen to family, encourage parents to assist with daily care of child, encourage parents to treat child as "normal," provide family with support group to discuss feelings, assess how each member is coping with stress and discuss healthier ways to cope as needed, give family as much control of child in hospital as possible, let family know you care.

c. **Interruptions in routines** — Assess patient's daily home routines (meals, voiding, play, school, baths), and attempt to incorporate into hospital care, allow as much independence and decision making as possible, discuss with child what would make hospitalization better for them.

d. **Interruption in school** — Utilize playroom or schoolroom and teachers as available, allow time for schoolwork, encourage reading, writing, and ask child questions pertaining to school, allow child to interact/play with other children their age, encourage visits, letters from schoolmates and teachers.

e. **Isolation** — Utilize washable toys, books, television, telephone, coloring books in room, explain necessity of isolation and length, encourage visits by parents; talk to, touch and spend time with child, play games or other activities which promote interaction.

f. **Loneliness** — Prevent by introducing child to others in age group, allow child to go to playroom, encourage utilization of telephone, writing letters, provide as much interaction as possible, allow child to discuss feelings and suggest ways that might help them cope with the loneliness.

g. **Pain** — Assess location, frequency, duration, and cause, differentiate between physiological and psychological pain, use pain scales such as Wong-Baker faces, numerical analog, or pain thermometer. Always assess effectiveness of pain medications.

- **Infants** — Will display change in vital signs, and withdrawal of area in pain; administer medications as ordered; reposition, stroke, swaddle, rock, talk to; infants unable to localize and communicate where discomfort is; determine and record effectiveness of interventions

- **Toddlers** — Will display change in vital signs, have child point to and describe pain, utilize a face scale to monitor degree of pain and how child feels, document location and degree of pain and alleviating activities, medicate as ordered, hold, reposition, allow play and movement, determine and record effectiveness of interventions
- **Preschoolers** — Will display change in vital signs, have child identify site and intensity or sensation, what would make them feel better, evaluate using face scale, utilize repositioning, distraction, imagery and pain medications as needed, hold/stroke child, keep environment quiet and non-threatening, allow play and movement, determine and record effectiveness of interventions
- **Schoolage** — Have child identify site and intensity, assess pain using a rating scale (0-10), or other descriptive pain scale, reposition, utilize imagery, distractions, pain medication as needed, determine and record effectiveness of intervention
- **Adolescents** — Have patient identify site, intensity, duration and sensation, utilize repositioning, imagery, distraction and pain medication as ordered, determine and record effectiveness of interventions

h. **Restraints** — Provide 10 minutes each hour in which movement is allowed, maintain movement in as many extremities as possible, provide age-appropriate stimulation:

- **Infants:** Mobiles, busy box, tapes, touching, rocking
- **Toddlers:** Busy boxes, noise makers, allow to walk every hour when awake
- **Preschoolers, schoolage, and adolescents:** Explain need for restraints, length of use, and limitation; provide colors, TV, books, musical instruments, and interaction as diversionary activities

i. **Restricted diet/NPO** — Continue thorough mouth care, discourage parent from bringing in food or eating in front of child, limit discussion of food, provide other activities during regular mealtime, discuss length and limitations of food/fluid restrictions.

VI. Play Therapy

1. Play room should be a safe haven, no procedures should be performed in this area.

2. Play should be a part of every child's daily routines.

3. Play is an excellent outlet for childhood anxiety and energy.

4. Play should be age-appropriate and meet safety requirements.

5. Play should be brought to the room for children in isolation.

VII. Discharge Planning

1. The nurse should begin preparing the parent and child for discharge, beginning on the day of admission.

2. Discharge planning should be a daily progression so that the family and child are prepared to go home when the physician discharges the child.

3. Items to include in making an assessment for discharge:
   a. Physical needs at home
   b. Ability to perform ADLs
   c. Home and school environment
   d. Special care needs (medication administration, PT, OT)
   e. Special nutritional requirements
   f. Psychological needs of child and family
   g. Learning needs of child and family
   h. Family's ability to care for child once discharged

4. Items to include in teaching:
   a. Explanation of disorder
   b. Specific care required for disorder
   c. Correct medication administration (drug, dose, route, time and side effects)
   d. Signs and symptoms which require parents to seek medical attention
   e. Phone number to call to seek medical attention
   f. How to get help in case of emergency
   g. Date of next follow-up appointment

3

RESPIRATORY DISORDERS

I.   General Concepts

- The respiratory system is composed of the oropharynx, nasopharynx, larynx, trachea, bronchi, bronchioles, lungs and alveoli

- The pediatric respiratory system continues to mature after birth

- The infant's respiratory tract is more susceptible to obstruction than the adult's due to these differences in anatomy: greater soft palate, larger tongue, larger amounts of soft tissue in airway; these anatomical differences predispose infants to greater risk of obstruction if airway becomes swollen; alveoli continue to mature after birth

- Infants are nose breathers and utilize the diaphragm to breathe; therefore, nasal obstruction can cause anoxia in infancy

- Signs that indicate respiratory difficulty include: coughing, wheezing, rhinorrhea, irritability or nervousness, tachypnea; as severity progresses respiratory distress may occur and is recognized by anxiety, nasal flaring, use of accessory muscles for respiration, (causing retractions), paleness, cyanosis, grunting, tachycardia, irritability; prompt treatment is required to prevent respiratory collapse and failure

- Whether disorders are acute or chronic, they may be life threatening, and require prompt treatment

II. Specific Respiratory Disorders

Congenital Defects

1. CYSTIC FIBROSIS (CF)

a. **Description** — An autosomal recessive disorder in which there is over-production of mucous by the exocrine glands. The excess viscous mucous affects the lungs, small intestines, pancreas and bile ducts. It is a progressive disease process which eventually leads to an early death, usually by late twenties. It is the number one cause of genetically-related deaths in Caucasian children.

b. **Signs and Symptoms** — Symptoms may or may not be present initially. Pulmonary signs include coughing, tachypnea, retractions (infancy), bronchial plugging, pneumothorax, increased number of respiratory infections, pulmonary function tests that indicate increased residual volume, increased total lung capacity, decreased vital capacity and decreased flow rates, dyspnea, wheezing, atelectasis, productive coughing. Gastrointestinal signs include: meconium ileus (newborn), loose stools, poor weight gain, chronic diarrhea, voracious appetite, abdominal distension, prolapse of rectum, intestinal obstruction, steatorrhea, azotorrhea, pancreatic insufficiency, gastroesophageal reflux, gallstones.

c. **Diagnostic Procedures** — Pilocarpine iontophoresis for sweat electrolytes reveals chloride greater than 60mg/L, pancreatic enzyme evaluation shows decreased levels present, fat absorption assessment reveals diminished fat absorption present, and family history positive for CF. Pulmonary function tests (PFTs) are helpful in determining pulmonary changes.

d. **Medical Interventions**

  – **Medications** — Administration of pancreatic enzymes, bronchodilators, long-term suppressive antibiotic therapy, increased salt intake, DNase (recombinant human deoxyribonuclease); recombinant human growth hormone is being evaluated as to the effectiveness of increasing strength and endurance; nasal cromolyn sodium, corticosteroids and occasional use of nasal decongestants can help nasal polyps; yearly vaccination against influenza; laxatives, stool softeners to decrease constipation and meconiumileus

  – **Treatments** — Maintain healthy pulmonary functioning (CPT, hydration, pulmonary hygiene); provide diet which is 130-150% greater than normal caloric needs with fat content 30% of total calories; adequate salt intake; provide multivitamins, vitamin E, K, D, and calcium

  – **Surgery** — Surgical pleurodesis, partial pleurectomy, surgical removal of nasal polyps, bronchoscopy to cauterize or ambolize bleeding, lung transplants

e. Nursing Interventions
 – **Assessment and Actions**
   * Assess child's respiratory and nutritional status
   * Monitor child's weight and growth parameters frequently
   * During hospitalization monitor vital signs, respiratory status, hydration status, comfort level, and prevent further infections
   * Ensure respiratory treatments are done
   * Encourage healthy diet
   * Administer medications as ordered
   * Encourage exercise (swimming, walking, jogging) and alternate with rest periods at home
   * Assess for signs indicating potential complications (e.g., clubbing, decreased PFTs, infection, decreased or congested lung sounds, fatigue, weight loss, change in stools)
   * Refer parents to genetic counseling
   * If patient is an adolescent or young adult, refer for genetic counseling and information regarding family planning
 – **Teaching**
   * Explain diagnosis to parent and child
   * Explain treatment regimen:
     1. Administer pancreatic enzymes regularly with meals to enhance absorption
     2. Provide high calorie, high protein foods in diet, as well as vitamin supplements
     3. Encourage liberal use of salt on foods and electrolyte fluids when febrile, during hot weather, and with physical exertion
     4. Monitor child's weight weekly
   * Teach parents and child CPT, postural drainage, oxygen therapy and positioning to promote clearing of lung fields; encourage fluid intake prior to treatment to loosen secretions
   * Instruct child in breathing exercise and assist with selecting regular times to perform
   * Teach parent and child about medications prescribed (drug, dose, route, time, and side effects) and how to use inhaler
   * Teach parents how to give intravenous medications and care of central lines if home care
 – **Emotional Care**
   * Promote growth and development and encourage child to do as much for self as possible
   * Discuss chronicity of disease and how child and family are coping
   * Provide emotional support to family and child, refer for possible counseling

* Provide support group information to family (national and local Cystic Fibrosis Foundation)

f. **Potential Complications** — Malabsorption syndrome, emphysema, rectal prolapse, cirrhosis, portal hypertension, respiratory infections, spontaneous pneumothorax, death.

Acquired Defects

1. **ASTHMA (BRONCHIAL)**

a. **Description** — A reversible, obstructive airway disease associated with airway irritability and bronchospasm, which causes trapping of air in the bronchioles. It may be intermittent or chronic and may be due to an allergic reaction or have a genetic link. It leads to respiratory acidosis if left untreated. It is often the great imitator of other disease processes and, therefore, it is important to rule out: foreign-body obstruction, cystic fibrosis, congestive heart failure, laryngotracheal malacia, and vocal cord paresis before diagnosis is confirmed. It is the most common illness in childhood and is responsible for more missed school days than any other illness.

b. **Signs and Symptoms** — Acute or gradual onset of expiratory wheezing, chest tightness, retractions, tachypnea, nonproductive coughing with or without wheezing, cyanosis, diaphoresis, nervousness, altered mental status; child may position self over table or chair leaning forward to ease respiratory efforts.

c. **Diagnostic Procedures** — Diagnosed by history, physical findings, presence of elevated pCO_2, CXR usually not helpful unless to rule out obstruction, sweat chloride test utilized to rule out CF, immunological assay tests reveal elevated IgE, pulmonary function test utilized to determine degree of lung disease and response to therapy. Spirometry and peak expiratory flow rate (PEFR) used as indicators for medications and response to treatment.

d. **Medical Interventions**

– **Medications** — Administer oxygen, bronchodilators, epinephrine, albuterol, theophylline, terbutaline, ipratropium bromide, salmeterol xinafoate; anti-inflammatory agents such as cromolyn sodium, medocromil; glucocorticoids (parenteral, oral and inhaled); antibiotics for infections. New asthma medications such as leukotriene synthesis inhibitors and receptor antagonist, 5-lipoxygenase inhibitors, and anti-Ig E antibody are being developed

– **Treatments** — Identify and remove causative agent, improve pulmonary function by medication, teach breathing exercises, increase hydration by IV, maintain normal lifestyle and promote exercise

– **Surgery** — Unnecessary

e. **Nursing Interventions**

– **Assessment and Actions**

* Assess and evaluate level of distress and position child for comfort and to facilitate breathing

* Monitor vital signs
* Assist child and family in identifying early warning signs of attack (itchy throat, "funny" feeling in chest, nervousness, paleness) and to take immediate action, including medication administration, positioning child to enhance breathing, promote rest and fluids
* Monitor child for therapeutic response and/or untoward effects of medication
* Assess and monitor child's environment and remove or decrease causative agents/situations
* Assess for signs indicating potential complications (sudden decrease in wheezing, drop in PaO_2 or increase in $PaCO_2$, downward trend in oxygen saturations)
* Assist child and family in identifying "triggers" or causative agents or situations that precipitate or aggravate asthma symptoms (stress, allergies, upper respiratory infections, air pollution, irritants such as tobacco, cleaning agents, exercise, cold air, gastroesophageal reflux, etc.)

- **Teaching**
  * Explain diagnosis to parent and child
  * Prepare child and family for treatment regimen (medication administration, oxygen therapy, rehydration) and instruct on importance of each
  * Teach parents and child correct use of metered dose inhaler and spacers and obtain return demonstration; discuss when to use inhaler and action to take if relief not obtained after use
  * Teach child breathing exercises to extend expiratory time and increase expiratory effort
  * Teach parent about medication prescribed (drug, dose, route, time, and side effects); instruct that the medication regimen is very strict and medications must be given exactly as prescribed
  * Teach child and family the correct use of the peak flow meter to obtain PEFR
  * Emphasize to parents the importance of prompt treatment when an attack occurs

- **Emotional Care**
  * Promote normal growth and development
  * Provide support to family and child
  * Provide support group information to family

f. **Potential Complications** — Infection, collapsed lung, emphysema, atelectasis, status asthmaticus (the body's inability to respond to the treatment regimen for asthma). This condition requires emergency treatment. Signs of respiratory distress increase and metabolic acidosis occurs; treatment focuses on administration of IV epinephrine, aminophylline, corticosteroids, oxygen therapy, IV fluids, resuscitation, treatment of acidosis, monitoring vital signs and providing support to family and child. This can be fatal if not treated.

2. **BRONCHIOLITIS**

   a. **Description** — An inflammation of the bronchioles accompanied by mucous obstruction. It is often caused by the respiratory synctial virus and affects children less than two years of age. It can be fatal if left untreated.

   b. **Signs and Symptoms** — Usually acute in onset, history of upper respiratory infection for several days, rhinorrhea, shallow respirations, dry, harsh, cough, retractions, cyanosis, fever, crackles, grunting, nasal flaring, expiratory wheezes, loss of appetite, tachypnea, diminished breath sounds and atelectasis on auscultation; may be associated with otitis media and/or pneumonia.

   c. **Diagnostic Procedures** — Diagnosis is determined by physical findings, presence of hyperinflation of lungs, retractions, ruling out asthma, as well as obtaining a positive culture for the respiratory syncitial virus (RSV).

   d. **Medical Interventions**

      – **Medications** — Administer bronchodilators (may not be effective in 50% of the cases), epinephrine, oral steroids, Ribavirin (only if RSV infection confirmed), RSV immune globulin for high risk children (CF, BPD, chronic lung disease)

      – **Treatments** — Maintain airway, prevent secondary infection, administer oxygen, fluids, and perform intubation if severe symptoms present; hospitalization may be required if dehydration, secondary bacterial infection or respiratory distress occur

      – **Surgery** — Unnecessary

   e. **Nursing Interventions**

      – **Assessment and Actions**

         * Assess child's vital signs, hydration status, and be alert for increasing signs of respiratory distress
         * Administer medications, oxygen (via nasal cannula, oxygen hood or ET tube), fluids, increased humidity
         * Maintain quiet environment
         * Keep child in contact isolation and utilize thorough handwashing
         * Assess for signs indicating potential complications

      – **Teaching**

         * Explain diagnosis and treatment regimen to parents
         * Teach parents about medication prescribed (drug, dose, route, time and side effects)
         * Teach parents about isolation and handwashing; emphasize necessity in following isolation regimen; instruct that this limits spread of RSV to others as it is not as fragile as other viruses

and may live up to 48 hours on inanimate objects such as clothing

- **Emotional Care**
    * Promote growth and development while hospitalized
    * Provide support to parents and child
f. **Potential Complications** — Secondary respiratory infection, hypoxia, death (in severe untreated cases).

3. **BRONCHOPULMONARY DYSPLASIA (BPD)**

   a. **Description** — A chronic lung disorder in which there is hypertrophy of small airways, squamous metaplasia and fibrosis of the alveoli and bronchioles. The alveoli collapse and air movement is trapped. It occurs in infants who require prolonged mechanical ventilation with high oxygen tensions (increased PIP), meconium aspiration syndrome, persistent pulmonary hypertension, pneumonia, and cyanotic heart disease.

   b. **Signs and Symptoms** — Signs of respiratory distress, tachypnea, tachycardia, cyanosis on room air, long-term oxygen dependency, growth and developmental delays, difficulty feeding, barrel-chest appearance (in long-term disorder), inability to wean from mechanical ventilation.

   c. **Diagnostic Procedures** — Diagnosed by birth history, x-ray reveals hyperaeration and atelectasis, ABG reveals hypoxia or compensating hypercarbia, acidosis, and mild hypoxemia; echocardiogram shows right ventricular hypertrophy.

   d. **Medical Interventions**
      - **Medications** — Administer oxygen, theophylline, terbutaline, isoproterenol, diuretics, steroids, surfactant replacement therapy (at delivery in preterm infants)
      - **Treatments** — Monitor oxygenation using transcutaneous PaO_2, provide positive pressure ventilation, increase nutritional intake, and maintain hydration status
      - **Surgery** — Unnecessary

   e. **Nursing Interventions**
      - **Assessment and Actions**
          * Assess child's vital signs, respiratory, hydration, electrolyte and nutritional status; assess carefully for signs and symptoms of viral respiratory infections (chronically-ill infants have increased susceptibility)
          * Be prepared for intubation
          * Prepare parents for long-term therapy (usually resolves by 3-4 years)
          * Assess signs indicating potential complications
      - **Teaching**
          * Explain diagnosis and treatment regimen to family

* Prepare for home care by teaching signs of respiratory distress to parents and teaching them when to seek medical help, and how to adminsiter CPR
* Teach parents about medications prescribed (drug, dose, route, time and side effects)
* Teach signs and symptoms of infection and to avoid contact with persons with known infections

– **Emotional Care**

* Promote growth and development and promote rest
* Provide support to family and child

f. **Potential Complications** — Infection, congestive heart failure, respiratory failure, pneumothorax, chronic respiratory disease (life-long), long-term developmental and growth retardation, death.

4. **EPIGLOTTITIS (ACUTE)**

a. **Description** — A bacterial infection of the epiglottis causing edema and inflammation. It is a rapidly progressing disorder and is a medical emergency. It must be treated promptly before complete airway obstruction occurs. This disorder is typically seen among children 2-5 years old but can occur at any age. It is most commonly caused by *H. influenza* Type B.

b. **Signs and Symptoms** — Initial onset may be quite subtle with increasing restlessness. As the condition progresses, signs and symptoms include: inspiratory stridor, high fever, muffled voice, barking cough, sore throat. If untreated, inspiratory stridor, tachypnea, fear, retractions, dysphagia, excessive drooling, respiratory distress and obstruction occur. Typically child assumes a "tripod" position supporting body with hands with chin thrust forward and mouth open in attempt to open airway wider.

c. **Diagnostic Procedures** — Diagnosed by physical assessment, lateral x-ray reveals enlarged or thumb-like epiglottis. Quick ventilation may be required via intubation, then, the swollen, cherry red epiglottis can be seen. Inspection of the epiglottis should be performed only when intubation and emergency tracheostomy equipment is available.

d. **Medical Interventions**

– **Medications** — Administer antibiotics (Deftriaxone, ampicillin and sulbactum, corticosteroids). Administration of H. influenzae vaccine can prevent the disease

– **Treatments** — Maintain open airway by artificial airway placement and provide fluid resuscitation as needed. Prepare to intubate

– **Surgery** — Tracheostomy may be necessary, especially if intubation is not possible

e. Nursing Interventions
- **Assessment and Actions**
  * Be alert to signs and symptoms and treat promptly
  * Position child for comfort and safety
  * Assist with intubation or tracheostomy and secure tube
  * Assess vital signs, hydration status, ABGs, comfort level
  * Administer antibiotics as ordered
  * Determine method in which child can communicate
  * Once extubated, monitor respiratory status and offer fluids
  * Assess for signs indicating potential complications
- **Teaching**
  * Explain diagnosis and need for emergency treatment
  * Teach parents about medications prescribed (drug, dose, route, time, and side effects)
- **Emotional Care**
  * Encourage parents to remain with child until child is calm
  * Provide support to family and child and reassure that treatment is focused on reducing the size of the epiglottis and maintaining airway function

f. Potential Complications — Death from occlusion of airway.

5. FOREIGN BODY ASPIRATION (FBA)

a. Description — A partial or complete blockage of the airway. It is typically seen in infants and toddlers. It may be life threatening and is often due to ingestion of small items (raisins, peanuts, gum, popcorn, hot dog).

b. Signs and Symptoms — Depends on whether partial or complete obstruction has occurred and on location; partial obstruction symptoms include choking, coughing, wheezing, gagging, whistling sound on inspiration, diminished breath sounds or chest movement on affected side retractions, cyanosis; complete obstruction of upper airway causes absence of breathing, nervousness, fainting, severe cyanosis and eventual death, if left untreated.

c. Diagnostic Procedures — Diagnosed by history, physical examination, x-ray reveals lodged item or trapped air, bronchoscopy may be used to visualize, confirm, or retrieve item.

d. Medical Interventions
- **Medications** — Administer oxygen and antibiotics after removal
- **Treatments** — Partial obstruction requires removal by bronchoscopy or laryngoscopy; complete obstruction requires the Heimlich Maneuver or emergency intubation
- **Surgery** — Tracheostomy placement may be necessary to open airway

e. **Nursing Interventions**
   – **Assessment and Actions**
     * Assist with prompt diagnosis and administer emergency treatment
     * Prepare child for sedation and anesthesia if bronchoscopy or laryngoscopy required
     * Describe necessity of tracheostomy to parents and what to expect if tracheostomy placement required
     * Assess vital signs, respiratory status, keep environment calm, keep patient NPO initially after removal of object
     * Avoid treatments or activities which may cause further irritation to respiratory system (CPT, coughing)
     * Assess for signs indicating potential complications (increased respiratory distress, unable to cry or speak, cyanosis, collapse)
   – **Teaching**
     * Explain diagnosis to parents and discuss treatment required
     * Discuss safety in home and identify appropriate items to allow child to play with; eliminate potential hazards such as balloons, hot dogs, peanut butter, toys with small removable parts, etc.)
     * Teach parents CPR before discharged
     * Teach parents about medication prescribed (drug, dose, route, time, and side effects)
   – **Emotional Care**
     * Provide support to family and child
     * Provide time for grieving and refer to counseling if death occurs
f. **Potential Complications** — Swelling of airway after removal, erosion of airway if undetected initially, infection, if hypoxic for several minutes may cause brain damage and/or death.

6. **LARYNGOTRACHEOBRONCHITIS (LTB)**
   a. **Description** — A viral respiratory infection that has a slowly progressive onset. It causes inflammation and swelling of the laryngeal area and usually occurs in the toddler age group. It is the most common form of croup and is more common in boys than girls. It is most commonly caused by parainfluenza 1,2, and 3 viruses, respiratory syncytial virus, and rhinovirus.

   b. **Signs and Symptoms** — Symptoms occur more commonly at night and during cold seasons. History of upper respiratory infection, hoarseness, barking cough, retractions, inspiratory stridor, diminished breath sounds, mild fever, crackles, rhonchi, cyanosis, tachycardia, nervousness; differentiated from acute spasmodic croup by slower, more gradual onset.

   c. **Diagnostic Procedures** — Diagnosed by reviewing history, ruling out epiglottitis by lateral neck x-ray; visual inspection reveals subglottal narrowing.

d. Medical Interventions

- **Medications** — Administer corticosteroids, nebulized racemic epinephrine if hospitalized, Ribavarin (only if RSV infection confirmed), antibiotics if secondary bacterial infection (i.e., otitis media) present
- **Treatments** — Maintain airway, provide humidified oxygen, monitor for continued airway difficulty and distress, rehydrate, may require intubation if symptoms not relieved
- **Surgery** — Unnecessary

e. Nursing Interventions

- **Assessment and Actions**
  * Assist with prompt diagnosis
  * If hospitalized, assess vital signs, respiratory efforts and for progressive worsening; monitor I & O, have intubation equipment at hand, administer mist oxygen as ordered and monitor oxygenation
  * Keep child calm, generally held by parent to decrease child's distress
  * Assess for signs indicating potential complications
- **Teaching**
  * Explain diagnosis to parents and discuss treatment regimen
  * If child treated at home, discuss with parents signs of increasing respiratory difficulty and when to seek further medical assistance; encourage using humidifier and keeping child quiet in bed
  * Instruct parents to offer fluids liberally unless potential for aspiration
  * Prepare parents for coughing or vomiting of mucous after crises resolved
  * Teach parents about medication prescribed (drug, dose, route, time, and side effects)
- **Emotional Care**
  * Provide quiet activities in bed appropriate for age
  * Encourage parents to stay with child and instruct them to keep child under tent if hospitalized
  * Provide support to family and child

f. Potential Complications — Recurrence, infection, death if severe and untreated.

7. RESPIRATORY DISTRESS SYNDROME (RDS)

a. Description — A progression in alveolar insufficiency and collapse that causes atelectasis, hypoxemia, and respiratory compromise. It is seen in preterm infants and is due to insufficient surfactant production. It was previously know as hyaline membrane disease (HMD).

b. **Signs and Symptoms** — Initially at birth symptoms absent but infant quickly (30 minutes to 2 hours postdelivery) exhibits respiratory symptoms: retractions, nasal flaring, tachypnea, grunting, cyanosis, apnea while on room air; leads to metabolic and respiratory acidosis.

c. **Diagnostic Procedures** — Diagnosed by history, ABGs reveals increased CO_2, and x-ray of lung field which shows atelectasis (ground-glass appearance) and air-filled bronchioles.

d. **Medical Interventions**

   – **Medications** — Administer oxygen via artificial airway (ET tube, nasal prongs) prn, administer replacement surfactant at delivery as prophylaxis for RDS or later as rescue treatment; may administer pharmacological paralyzing agents (pancuronium or vecuronium) and sedative agents (morphine sulfate, ativan, fentanyl, and demerol); antenatal administration of corticosteroid to mother may stimulate production of surfactant; broad spectrum antibiotics (ampicillin and gentamicin) used until sepsis ruled out

   – **Treatments** — Maintain respiratory function, correct acidosis, prevent complications, provide sedation, monitor nutrition and fluid status

   – **Surgery** — May be necessary to correct a patent ductus arteriosus (PDA) which has not closed after delivery and causes a left to right shunting of blood from aorta to pulmonary arteries thus prolonging respiratory problems

e. **Nursing Interventions**

   – **Assessment and Actions**

      * Assess preterm infant after birth for respiratory problems and obtain prompt interventions from physician

      * Monitor administration of oxygen and maintain airway

      * Assess vital signs, respiratory status

      * Maintain neutral thermal environment to decrease metabolic requirements

      * Maintain minimal stimulation policy (quiet environment, low lighting, minimal handling)

      * Monitor for signs and symptoms of PDA ("washing machine" murmur, bounding peripheral pulses, increased oxygen/respiratory support demands, and decreased ability to wean from respiratory support)

      * Assess nutritional needs and monitor growth pattern

      * Provide appropriate developmental intervention as infant's condition allows

      * Encourage parental participation in care and decision making

      * Monitor carefully for signs and symptoms of infection and oxygen toxicity

      * Assess for signs indicating potential complications

      * If mother planning to breastfeed, encourage her to utilize a breast pump until infant's status improves

- **Teaching**
  * Discuss diagnosis and treatment regimen with family
  * Prepare family for what to expect child to look like (monitors, tubing, IV sites, sounds)
- **Emotional Care**
  * Provide support to family and child
  * Promote bonding
  * Allow parents to visit as much as possible

  f. **Potential Complications** — BPD, infections, retinopathy of prematurity (damage to the retina due to excessive oxygenation), intraventricular hemorrhage, pneumothorax, pulmonary interstitial emphysema (PIE), pneumopericardium, vena cava syndrome (due to increased pressure in thorax that decreases blood return to heart), necrotizing enterocolitis (NEC), death.

8. **PNEUMONIA**

  a. **Description** — A viral or bacterial pulmonary infection occurring frequently in infancy and early childhood. It may be a primary disease or be the result of another illness. It is manifested by inflammation and consolidation of pulmonary parenchyma. It is classified by the causative agent with viral being more common (most often respiratory syncytial virus). The bacterial form is caused most often by pneumococci, streptococci, staphylococci, chlamydia or mycoplasma. Pneumococcal is most often spread by respiratory droplet in winter and early spring; chlamydial is severe, diffuse and often difficult to treat; staphylococcal often is the primary infection (usually nosocomial in origin); and, streptococcal lobular, less common, is spread via the lymphatic system.

  b. **Signs and Symptoms** — Viral: acute or insidious onset, slight or severe cough, slow to high grade fever, malaise to lethargy. Bacterial: abrupt onset, lethargy, preceded by viral infection, respiratory distress, shocky appearance, decreased breath sounds, coarse crackles, friction rub, use of accessory muscles, nasal discharge. Mycoplasma: sudden or gradual fever, malaise, dry hacking cough, blood-tinged mucus, frequently seen in 5-12 year-olds. Chlamydia: usually 1-4 months of age in onset, persistent cough and tachypnea.

  c. **Diagnostic Procedures** — Viral: CXR reveals diffuse infiltrates; Bacterial: CXR shows patchy consolidation of one or more lobes, pneumatoceles (staph) or pleural effusions (strep), areas of consolidation (mycoplasma). White blood cell count increased in bacterial, normal or slightly decreased in viral.

  d. **Medical Interventions**
- **Medications** — Antibiotics specific for organism. Viral not treated with antibiotics unless secondary bacterial infection also present; antipyretics, IV fluid
- **Treatments** — Maintain patent airway, fever reduction, oxygen, pulmonary hygiene (CPT, updrafts), mist or humidity. Thoracen-

tesis may be necessary to obtain culture, to relieve fluid accumulation, and to administer antibiotics directly into the pleural cavity

  – **Surgery** — Unnecessary

e. **Nursing Interventions**

  – **Assessment and Actions**

  * Be alert to signs and symptoms of increasing respiratory distress/failure

  * Monitor for loss of patent airway

  * Assess vital signs, hydration status, ABGs, comfort level

  * Assess effectiveness of antibiotic and antipyretic therapy

  * Assess effectiveness of oxygen therapy

  * Assist with diagnostic procedures and maintenance of good pulmonary hygiene

  – **Teaching**

  * Explain meaning of diagnosis and planned medical treatment including all medications prescribed

  * Explain signs, symptoms and prevention of recurrence

  * Explain when to seek additional medical treatment (if not hospitalized)

  – **Emotional Care**

  * Encourage parents to remain with child

  * Provide support to child and family; assure parents that onset of pneumonia is often sudden and provide positive reinforcement for seeking care

f. **Potential Complications** — Secondary infection, respiratory failure, dehydration, febrile seizures, atelectasis, pulmonary abscesses, pneumothorax, death.

9. **TONSILLITIS (STREPTOCOCCAL PHARYNGITIS)**

  a. **Description** — An inflammation and formation of edema of the lymphoid tissue (tonsils) in the palatine or pharyngeal area of the mouth. It is frequently caused by Group A Beta hemolytic streptococci and is commonly seen in childhood.

  b. **Signs and Symptoms** — Reddened, swollen tonsils usually with exudate (may become so enlarged that they block passageway of air), sore throat, difficulty swallowing, hoarseness or muffling of voice, fever, lymphadenopathy, abdominal pain; may be accompanied by otitis media, sinusitis, skin rash or peritonsillar abscesses. May progress to meningitis, rheumatic fever, or acute glomerulonephritis.

  c. **Diagnostic Procedures** — Diagnosed by inspection and obtaining positive throat culture; ASO titer also increased late in the disease. History of streptococcus exposure.

d. Medical Interventions

- **Medications** — Administration of antibiotics (penicillin, cephalosporin, erythromycin or clindamycin) and antipyretics. Strep carrier may require penicillin and refampin

- **Treatments** — Promote gargling with warm salt water if mild, bedrest, increased fluid intake; if surgery required prevent sucking activity postoperatively

- **Surgery** — Surgical removal of tonsils if blocking airway or if recurrent inflammation occurs (tonsillectomy)

e. Nursing Interventions

- **Assessment and Actions**

  * Assist with obtaining throat culture

  * Assess vital signs, hydration status, and comfort level

  * Position patient prone or on side postoperatively to prevent pooling of blood in back of throat

  * Assess for signs of hemorrhage postoperatively (frequent swallowing, vomiting frank blood, pallor)

  * Prevent irritation to surgical area (prevent coughing, avoid use of straw, serve only bland foods when off NPO status)

  * Promote oral hydration postoperatively by offering cool drinks, jello, ice chips, nonacidic drinks

  * Encourage high fluid intake to prevent crusting of incision — if wound crusts over and breaks off, hemorrhage can occur

  * Provide method for reducing discomfort (warm or cool compress to throat/neck)

  * Assess for signs indicating potential complications (bleeding postop, respiratory distress)

- **Teaching**

  * Discuss diagnosis and treatment regimen with parents and child

  * If home care prescribed, discuss with parents antibiotic administration, antipyretic administration, increasing fluid intake of cool nonacidic liquids, gargling with warm salt water, utilizing vaporizor, isolation and handwashing

  * If tonsillectomy required, prepare child and family for procedure and postoperative care

  * Prepare family and child for discharge after surgery (omit sucking, spicy or hot foods or fluids) and teach them signs that would indicate bleeding

- **Emotional Care**

  * Provide support to family

f. Potential Complications — Postoperative hemorrhaging, occlusion of airway if severe edema develops. Untreated strep infections can lead to rheumatic fever, acute nephritis syndrome, tonsillar hypertrophy and sleep apnea.

CARDIOVASCULAR DISORDERS

I.   General Concepts

- The heart is completely formed by the eighth week of fetal development

- The heart is composed of four chambers: 2 atria and 2 ventricles, and four valves: tricuspid, mitral, aortic and pulmonic

- At birth, once the umbilical cord is clamped off, the pressure changes within the circulatory system causing the heart to begin functioning independently of maternal circulation

- The infant's heart is larger in proportion to the body than that of the adult's

- The heart grows throughout childhood and reaches adult size by the end of adolescence

- Pressure in the normal heart is greater on the left side than on the right

- Heart defects may be either congenital or acquired

II. Specific Cardiovascular Disorders

Congenital Heart Defects

- Cardiac defects that exist from birth

- May be undetected or life threatening depending upon the nature of the defect

- May be caused by maternal illness, maternal drug ingestion, maternal age (over 40), hereditary factors, or unknown etiology

- May be accompanied by other defects

- May cause: increased cardiac workload, pulmonary hypertension, diminished cardiac output, hypoxemia, cardiomegaly, altered growth and development, decreased activity tolerance, tachypnea, clubbing of fingers and toes, poor weight gain, poor feeding, cyanosis, diaphoresis

- May be so severe or damaging that a heart transplant is necessary

- Are categorized as acyanotic or cyanotic

Acyanotic Defects

Cardiac defects in which only, or predominantly, oxygenated blood enters the arterial circulation. The pressure on the left side of the heart is higher and allows the flow of blood to be shunted from the left to the right chambers. Cardiomegaly and pulmonary artery hypertrophy are commonly seen with this type of defect. The more commonly seen acyanotic defects include:

1. **ATRIAL SEPTAL DEFECT (ASD)**

    a. **Description** — The presence of an opening in the atrial septum. It may be due to the failure of the foramen ovale to close. Defects in this region of the atrial septum account for 9-10% of all lesions. Blood flows across the defect from left (high pressure) to right (low pressure) and causes increased pulmonary blood flow. The increased volume and workload result in right-sided hypertrophy and possibly mild to moderate pulmonary edema. This defect is seen more frequently in females.

    b. **Signs and Symptoms** — Usually asymptomatic; may have audible systolic ejection murmur at left sternal border; mild exercise intolerance; mild to moderate cardiomegaly with pulmonary vascular disease gradually increasing.

    c. **Diagnostic Procedures** — ECG may reveal atrial arrhythmias (prolonged P-R interval) and RVH; CXR reveals pulmonary vasculature, prominent pulmonary artery and right ventricular hypertrophy (RVH); echocardiogram reveals abnormal septal motion, dilated right atrium and right ventricle; angiography shows ASD; cardiac catheterization reveals increased O_2 saturations in right atrium.

   d. **Medical Interventions**
- **Medications** — Administer digitalis and diuretics if right or left ventricular failure occur; administer antibiotics postoperatively
- **Treatments** — May close spontaneously; monitor for signs of complications; transvenous closure in the catheterization lab with an occluding device is an alternative to surgical closure
- **Surgery** — Surgical repair may be performed if: defect is large with a large left-to-right shunt, congestive heart failure, or pulmonary congestion; females should always undergo surgical repair due to the high risk of paradoxical emboli in pregnancy

   e. **Nursing Interventions**
- See section on "Nursing Interventions," page 43

   f. **Potential Complications** — In adulthood: atrial arrhythmias, emboli, heart failure, left ventricular failure if uncorrected.

2. **COARCTATION OF THE AORTA**

   a. **Description** — The presence of a narrowing anywhere along the aortic arch. This narrowing causes decreased blood flow distal to the structure, and the back-up of blood flow in the heart. This defect is seen more frequently in males and is commonly seen in association with Turner's Syndrome.

   b. **Signs and Symptoms** — Usually depend upon severity; may experience hypertension in arterial branches proximal to the defect and hypotension distal to the defect; may be asymptomatic until adolescence if narrowing of area is mild; may have systolic murmur audible on back near left upper side; may have discrepancy in femoral pulses (decreased/absent femoral and pedal pulses with a brachial femoral lag).

   c. **Diagnostic Procedures** — X-ray notes enlargement in portion of aorta proximal to stricture, cardiomegaly, and pulmonary edema; cardiac catheterization demonstrates location of defect; echocardiogram allows for visualization of coarctation site, dilated right ventricle and hypoplastic left ventricle.

   d. **Medical Interventions**
- **Medications** — Administer digitalis, dopamine, diuretics, oxygen, prostaglandin E (in newborns to keep ductus arteriosus open)
- **Treatment** — Provide fluid monitoring, renal monitoring, rest; treatment for congestive heart failure may be required; balloon angioplasty can be used as a primary nonsurgical intervention; percutaneous balloon angioplasty is used for residual postoperative coarctation gradients and for recoarctation occurrence
- **Surgery** — Surgical repair to resect the area and reanastomosis (subclavian flap aortoplasty) usually occurrs within the first two years of life; later surgical repair can occur if the defect is less severe

   e. **Nursing Interventions**
- See section on "Nursing Interventions," page 43

f. **Potential Complications** — Death from heart failure and renal shut-down preoperatively, infective endocarditis, renal failure postoperatively, recoarctation, death.

3. **ENDOCARDIAL CUSHION DEFECT (COMPLETE)**

   a. **Description** — The presence of a defect in the atrial septum and septal leaflets of the tricuspid and mitral valves. This results from failure to develop during the embryonic period. It presents as a wide spectrum of minor to major atrioventricular (AV) canals. With a complete defect, the patient has incomplete formation of mitral valve and tricuspid valves, ASD, and high ventricular septal defect. Blood flows through this opening and causes a mixing of oxygenated and unoxygenated blood. It also causes increased pulmonary blood flow. The severity of the defect varies. This defect is seen equally in both sexes. A higher incidence is seen in children with Downs Syndrome.

   b. **Signs and Symptoms** — May be asymptomatic at birth, may have audible systolic murmur and diastolic murmur, cyanosis upon exertion or crying, increased pulmonary congestion and edema, congestive heart failure, and delayed growth.

   c. **Diagnostic Procedures** — Diagnosed by physical findings; ECG reveals change in QRS axis and possible prolonged P-R interval; CXR reveals cardiomegaly and pulmonary vascular markings; echocardiogram allows for visualization of defects and shows communication between the 4 chambers of the heart; cardiac catheterization and angiography confirm the diagnosis.

   d. **Medical Interventions**
      - **Medications** — Administer digitalis, diuretics, antibiotics prophylactically
      - **Treatment** — Provide rest and monitor fluid status, prevent increased oxygen consumption
      - **Surgery** — Surgical repair of the atrial septum atrioventricular canal is performed; the child may also require valve replacement or pulmonary artery banding. These are usually done before 6-12 months of age

   e. **Nursing Interventions**
      - See section on "Nursing Interventions," page 43

   f. **Potential Complications** — Heart failure, mitral regurgitation, pulmonary hypertension and irreversible vascular obstruction disease, congestive heart failure, complete heart block, arrhythmias postoperatively, death.

4. **PATENT DUCTUS ARTERIOSUS (PDA)**

   a. **Description** — The presence of a passageway (ductus arteriosis) between the pulmonary and aortic circulation which persists after birth. This defect is caused by the failure of the fetal ductus arteriosis to close. The defect allows flow of blood from the aorta (high pressure) back into the pulmonary circulation (low pressure). It causes increased pulmonary blood flow, causing a left-to-right shunt. This defect often closes naturally by 6 months of age. The child may also have a VSD and/or coarctation of the aorta. This defect accounts for 12% of congenital heart defects and occurs in 20-60% of all premature infants. There is also an increased incidence at higher altitudes and females are affected twice as often as males. PDA is also one of the most common congenital cardiac anomalies associated with maternal rubella during pregnancy.

b. **Signs and Symptoms** — Typically present at birth; audible "washing machine" murmur at the left sternal border, may also have widened pulse pressures and bounding pulses; increased volume to the lungs may result in volume overload.

c. **Diagnostic Procedures** — Diagnosed by physical findings; CXR may appear normal if defect is small or may reveal left-sided cardiomegaly if defect is large; echocardiogram allows for direct visualization of defect; ECG normal if defect small, but indicates left ventricular hypertrophy if defect is large; cardiac catheterization reveals normal or increased pressures in the right ventricle and pulmonary artery.

d. **Medical Interventions**
   – **Medications** — Administer Indomethacin
   – **Treatment** — Monitor cardiac and pulmonary status, I&O; transvenous occlusion in catheterization lab can be done in older children
   – **Surgery** — If asymptomatic, surgical repair is usually not utilized until the child becomes older (1-2 years); if systomatic (inability to wean from supplemental oxygen), PDA is ligated or banded

e. **Nursing Interventions**
   – See section on "Nursing Interventions," page 43

f. **Potential Complications** — Before surgery: pulmonary edema, pneumonia, pulmonary or systemic emboli, pulmonary hypertension, congestive heart failure. Postoperatively: infective endocarditis, pneumothorax, death.

5. **PULMONARY STENOSIS (PS)**

a. **Description** — A narrowing of one or more sites at the entrance of the pulmonary artery. This defect causes a resistance to the pulmonary artery, decreased pulmonary blood flow, a resistance to blood flow and, therefore, abnormally high right ventricular pressure and right ventricular hypertrophy. The pulmonary valve abnormality is the most common. PS has a male predominance and is often seen in association with Noonan Syndrome.

b. **Signs and Symptoms** — May be asymptomatic, findings depend upon the severity of the defect but may include a systolic ejection murmur, pulmonic ejection click, systolic thrill, complaint of dyspnea, and fatigue; may also be cyanotic and experience right ventricular failure and low cardiac output.

   c. **Diagnostic Procedures** — X-ray and echocardiogram reveal enlarged right ventricle in moderate to severe PS; echocardiogram shows defect and thickened pulmonary valve; cardiac catheterization not necessary to confirm defect

   d. **Medical Interventions**

      – **Medications** — Digitalis, diuretics, prophylactic antibiotics if valve involvement present

      – **Treatment** — Balloon valvuloplasty during cardiac catheterization may be utilized to dilate area

      – **Surgery** — Surgical intervention is performed if symptoms are moderate to severe; surgeon may need to replace the pulmonic valve if it is involved (pulmonic valvuloplasty or complete excision of dysplastic valve)

   e. **Nursing Interventions**

      – See section on "Nursing Interventions," page 43

   f. **Potential Complications** — Congestive heart failure, low cardiac output, infective endocarditis, death.

6. **VENTRICULAR SEPTAL DEFECT (VSD)**

   a. **Description** — VSD is the most commonly seen of the cardiac defects (comprises 25%). It is an opening between the right and left ventricles. It causes increased pulmonary blood flow. It may be associated with other defects, or occur independently, and has a higher incidence in males. VSDs may be singular or multiple and are frequently associated with other cardiac defects and is the most common cardiac defect found in chromosomal abnormalities.

   b. **Signs and Symptoms** — Usually asymptomatic, loud pansystolic murmur may be present; if large defect, may exhibit decreased exercise tolerance, increased respiratory infections, delayed growth and development, congestive heart failure, left ventricular hypertrophy and pulmonary edema. If marked pulmonary hypertension occurs, a ventricular lift is present and cyanosis may occur.

   c. **Diagnostic Procedures** — Larger VSD defects are detected by CXR which shows enlarged left atrium and ventricle; echocardiogram reveals size and location of defect, ECG shows RVH with large lesions.

   d. **Medical Interventions**

      – **Medications** — Administer digitalis and diuretics if in congestive heart failure, and antibiotics prophylactically for prevention of sub-acute bacterial endocarditis (SBE)

      – **Treatment** — Spontaneous closure may occur if small

      – **Surgery** — Treatment depends upon the severity of the defect; surgical closure is performed if the VSD does not close spontaneously; if poor surgical risk, pulmonary artery banding may be done palliatively; recently, closure of defect is accomplished by placing occluding device into defect during cardiac catheterization

e. **Nursing Interventions**
- See section on "Nursing Interventions," page 43

f. **Potential Complications** — Congestive heart failure, pulmonary edema, respiratory infections, altered growth and development, death.

7. **HYPOPLASTIC LEFT HEART SYNDROME (HLHS)**

a. **Description** — HLHS occurs in 1.5% of children with congenital heart disease, and has a male predominance. It is 100% fatal without surgical intervention. It involves aortic and mitral atresia with a small, nonfunctional left ventricle. The right ventricle maintains both the pulmonary and systemic circulation.

b. **Signs and Symptoms** — Infants present in the first week of life with congestive heart failure, dyspnea, hepatomegaly, low cardiac output, and weak or absent peripheral pulses. S2 is single with an ejection click, and a systolic ejection murmur is heard at the left sternal border.

c. **Diagnostic Procedures** — The CXR shows cardiomegaly and interstitial pulmonary edema. The ECG shows RVH with absence of the left-sided forces and an absent Q wave and prominent P wave. The echo demonstrates the hypoplastic left ventricle and aorta.

d. **Medical Interventions**
- **Medications** — Medications for congestive heart failure and palliative treatment are needed until surgical intervention can be accomplished; a prostaglandin E1 is needed to maintain ductal patency
- **Treatment** — Surgical intervention is the only treatment available; management includes palliative treatment and support for patients and families
- **Surgery** — Palliative surgical repair (Norwood procedure which involves 2-3 stages) can be performed until a cardiac transplant can be accomplished

e. **Nursing Interventions**
- See section on "Nursing Interventions," page 43

f. **Potential Complications** — Death, rejection of organ transplant, permanent immunosuppressive therapy, delayed growth and development, congestive heart failure, chronic infections.

Cyanotic Defects

Cyanotic defects are defects in which unoxygenated blood mixes with some oxygenated blood in the heart. A large amount of unoxygenated blood then leaves the heart going into circulation. Cyanosis is determined by the presence of at least 4-5 grams of unsaturated hemoglobin in the capillary bed. If the child is anemic, cyanosis may not appear. Also, cyanotic infants are often ashen, not blue. These defects cause the blood to flow from the right to the left side of the heart. More commonly seen cyanotic defects include:

1. TETRALOGY OF FALLOT (TOF)

a. Description — This defect comprises 10% of all reported defects and is seen in both sexes. It causes decreased pulmonary blood flow and consists of 4 anomalies (each with varying severity):

  – Ventricular septal defect
  – Pulmonary stenosis
  – Overriding aorta
  – Right ventricular hypertrophy

b. Signs and Symptoms — The predominate findings are cyanosis (degree depends upon severity of pulmonary stenosis); hypoxic spells after 2 months of age; pansystolic murmur; clubbing of fingers and toes (if defect continues long-term without treatment); dyspnea with exertion; delay in growth and development; polycythemia; child will frequently take a squatting position after walking or playing to increase blood flow to the heart or may draw up the extremities when lying down. Cyanosis may not be present at birth and some children are acyanotic (pink tint).

c. Diagnostic Procedures - Diagnosed by physical findings; ABGs reveal hypoxemia and acidosis; echocardiogram allows for visualization of defect; CXR shows right atrial and ventricular hypertrophy, normal left atrium and ventricle and small main pulmonary artery giving heart a boot-shaped appearance; shows RVH and right axis deviation.

d. Medical Interventions

  – **Medications** — Administer oxygen, digitalis, diuretics, and antibiotics prophylactically (SBE), beta-adrenergic blockade by IV use of propanolol. IV methoxamine and phenylephrine increase systemic vascular resistance
  – **Treatment** — Limit activity, monitor I&O
  – **Surgery** — Surgical repair of the VSD and pulmonary stenosis is done according to severity of the symptoms (usually at 18 months). If underdeveloped pulmonary arteries are present, a systemic-to-pulmonary shunt is created (Blalock-Taussig procedure); there is a low mortality rate associated with this repair; cardiac medications may be administered before surgery to treat symptoms and after surgery to enhance the function of the heart; total surgical correction is done when the child is older and more pulmonary bloodflow is needed, usually within the first year of life

e. Nursing Interventions

  – See section on "Nursing Interventions," page 43

f. Potential Complications — Postoperative bleeding, congestive heart failure, heart block, death.

2. **TRANSPOSITION OF THE GREAT VESSELS (TGV)**

   a. **Description** — A defect in which the aorta arises from the right ventricle and the pulmonary artery arises from the left ventricle, i.e. the two great vessels are reversed. This reversal creates two independently functioning circulatory systems. The severity of the defect depends upon the amount of blood being mixed. Usually a patent foramen ovale and/or ventricular septal defect or PDA are present to maintain the infant's life after birth. The infant cannot survive unless these defects are present. This defect is seen more frequently in males and there may be a family history of diabetes.

   b. **Signs and Symptoms** — Cardinal sign is severe cyanosis; audible murmur from the VSD and ASD, congestive heart failure develops shortly after birth; difficulty in feeding. Cyanosis and hypoxia increase as fetal structures (ductus arteriosis and foramen ovale) close.

   c. **Diagnostic Procedures** — Diagnosed by physical findings; ABGs reveal hypoxemia and acidosis; labs reveal hypoglycemia, hypocalcemia, and polycythemia; CXR reveals cardiomegaly, egg-shaped heart silhouette; echocardiogram allows for visualization of defect.

   d. **Medical Interventions**
      - **Medications** — Administer prostaglandin E (PGE) (to keep foramen ovale open), digitalis, diuretics
      - **Treatment** — May be palliative or the defect may be corrected surgically; palliative treatment includes enlarging the other defects or making the necessary defects if not present (ASD or VSD); making a shunt to allow mixing of the blood thereby increasing oxygenated blood to flow into the circulation; correction metabolic acidosis, hypoglycemia, and hypocalcemia, administering oxygen
      - **Surgery** — Surgical correction usually takes place before 1 year of age. Arterial switch procedure is done at 1-2 weeks of age; multiple other surgical interventions required as the child grows

   e. **Nursing Interventions**
      - See section on "Nursing Interventions," page 43

   f. **Potential Complications** — Arrhythmias, pulmonary vascular obstructive disease, residual shunting, death.

Nursing Interventions For Congenital Defects

   a. **Assessment and Actions**
      - Be alert to signs and symptoms that may indicate a possible defect and make a thorough assessment of the infant/child using inspection, auscultation, and palpation
      - Assess child's vital signs, weight, hydration status, activity level, color, respiratory efforts, nutritional status, and activity level of comfort
      - Monitor cardiac functioning (vital signs, ECG, respiratory efforts, skin color and temperature, I&O) preoperatively

  – Postoperatively monitor level of comfort and provide method of reducing discomfort
  – Assess for signs indicating potential complications
  – Be alert to signs and symptoms of CHF: cyanosis, diaphoresis, tachypnea, dyspnea, retractions, orthopnea, edema, wheezing, tachycardia, gallop rhythm, decreased urinary output, anorexia, decreased blood pressure and pulses

b. **Teaching**
  – Assess family and child's level of understanding
  – Explain diagnosis to child and family
  – Instruct parents in feeding techniques to minimize fatigue
  – Teach parents signs and symptoms for which to be alert: cyanosis, edema, fatigue, feeding difficulties, rapid pulse, rapid respirations, respiratory distress, change in behavior
  – Prepare the child and family for procedures and treatments by explaining the information clearly, allowing time for questions, and utilizing pictures or written information as indicated
  – Inform family, as indicated, if child may be at higher risk for developing complications which may include:
    * Infection or pain postprocedure and/or postoperative
    * Congestive heart failure
    * Bacterial endocarditis
  – Inform parents of special limitations of child's activity according to defect and suggest ways to enhance growth and development
  – Teach family about medications child will receive before and after corrective repair; include name of drug, dose, times of administration, side effects, adverse reactions, and long-term side effects
  – Prepare for discharge by teaching parents: how to care for child after procedures or surgery; what activity limitations are indicated; signs and symptoms that require further medical attention; and, provide phone numbers if questions or problems arise

c. **Emotional Care**
  – Be prepared to assist the family in the grieving process
  – Acknowledge parental concerns and concerns of the child
  – Allow child to voice concerns and ask questions
  – Promote growth and development while hospitalized
  – Provide support to family and child
  – Provide support group information to family

Acquired Heart Defects

Acquired heart defects include those diseases which are caused by:

1) An infectious disease process
2) An autoimmune response
3) Environmental, heredity, or unknown etiologies

1. **BACTERIAL ENDOCARDITIS (BE)**

   a. **Description** — An infection of the heart valves and inner lining of the heart valves which usually occurs in children with congenital cardiac defects, cardiac injuries or cardiac repairs.

   b. **Signs and Symptoms** — Audible new murmur or change in existing murmur, anorexia, malaise, arthralgia, intermittent low grade fever, weight loss, petechiae, splinter hemorrhaging.

   c. **Diagnostic Procedures** — Diagnosed by history of previous cardiac defect or surgery; physical findings; CBC reveals anemia; presence of increased ESR; microscopic hematuria; echocardiogram reveals vegetative growth; blood cultures are positive for the organism; CXR shows cardiomegaly.

   d. **Medical Interventions**
      - **Medications** — Administer penicillin, or ampicillin, gentamicin, cloxacillin, amphotericin B, flucytosine, streptomycin for 4-6 weeks for specific organism
      - **Treatment** — Limit activity
      - **Surgery** — Valve replacement may be necessary if congestive heart failure develops, valve malfunctions, infection persists or relapse occurs

   e. **Nursing Interventions**
      - **Assessment and Actions**
        * Be alert to signs and symptoms of disorder
        * Preoperatively and postoperatively assess vital signs, I&O, skin temperature and color, level of comfort
        * Assess for signs indicating potential complications
      - **Teaching**
        * Instruct patient and family on methods of prevention via prophylactic treatment to high risk candidates, especially prior to visiting the dentist (e.g., PO or IV antibiotics prior to dental work or surgery)
        * Explain diagnosis to parent and child
        * Explain treatment regimen, length and purpose
        * Inform parents of signs and symptoms and who to contact; teach parents and child about medication prescribed (drug, dose, route, time and side effects)

- **Emotional Care**
  - * Discuss concerns that family and child have
  - * Provide support to family and child
- **f. Potential Complications** — Persistent infection, congestive heart failure, death.

2. **CONGESTIVE HEART FAILURE (CHF)**

- **a. Description** — A type of cardiac malfunction which causes a diminished amount of blood to be ejected into the systemic circulation. CHF usually does not occur in children unless another cardiac disorder precedes it. It may be either predominantly right-sided or left-sided failure of the heart muscle.
- **b. Signs and Symptoms** — Dyspnea, fatigue, weakness, poor feeding and growth, sweating, coughing, pallor, cyanosis, cardiomegaly, tachycardia, tachypnea, and edema.
- **c. Diagnostic Procedures** — Diagnosed by physical findings, CXR reveals cardiomegaly; echocardiogram assists with determining cause.
- **d. Medical Interventions**
  - **Medications** — Administer oxygen, sedation (morphine), diuretics and digoxin, ACE inhibitors (angiotension converting enzyme) such as captopril or enalapril
  - **Treatment** — Correct underlying cause and improve heart function and tissue oxygenation; restrict sodium and fluid intake; monitor I&O
  - **Surgery** — Unnecessary unless to correct underlying cause
- **e. Nursing Interventions**
  - **Assessment and Actions**
    - * Be alert for signs and symptoms of CHF
    - * If hospitalized, monitor vital signs, lung sounds, edema, daily weight, and assess nutritional status
    - * Administer medications on schedule
    - * Draw digoxin levels and serum electrolytes as ordered noting results
    - * Observe signs of digoxin toxicity (changes in ECG)
    - * Provide skin care and frequently turn patient to prevent skin breakdown
    - * Place in cardiac chair or infant chair, elevate head of bed
    - * Monitor BP before and after ACE inhibitors
    - * Administer humidified oxygen
    - * Assess for signs indicating potential complications such as change in SaO_2 saturation, signs of respiratory distress, sweating, increased fatigue, poor feeding

- Teaching
  * Discuss diagnosis and treatment plan with parent and child
  * Instruct parent and child on medication prescribed (drug, dose, route, time, and side effects)
  * Inform parents and child of signs of digitalis toxicity; signs and symptoms include nausea, vomiting, anorexia, and brady-cardia; dysrhythmias may also occur in severe cases
  * Encourage parents to have child rest as much as possible to decrease the heart's workload
  * Emphasize importance of adequate nutritional intake for child and instruct parents how to feed child to minimize fatigue
- Emotional Care
  * Discuss impact disease has had on child and family
  * Provide support to family and child
  * Provide support group information to family

f. **Potential Complications** — Digoxin toxicity, skin breakdown, respiratory infections, death.

3. **RHEUMATIC FEVER (ACUTE)**

   a. **Description** — Rheumatic fever is an inflammatory disease which can affect many body systems including the heart, joints, and subcutane-ous tissue. It is thought to commonly follow an upper respiratory in-fection (Group A streptococci). It may occur at any age but primarily affects middle to late childhood.

   b. **Signs and Symptoms**
   - **Findings include**:
     * Carditis with accompanying murmur, cardiomegaly, tachy-cardia, CHF, Aschoff bodies (lesions that cause scarring and fi-brosis of the cusps of the valves)
     * Polyarthritis — redness, swelling, pain, heat in multiple joints
     * Chorea (involuntary movements)
     * Erythema marginatum (macular rash on trunk and extremities)
     * Subcutaneous nodules in joints, scalp and spine
     * Other nonspecific findings which may include anorexia, low-grade fever, and fatigue

   c. **Diagnostic Procedures** — Diagnosis is made by utilizing Jones criteria; a positive result is based on evidence of two major, or one major and two minor, criteria with positive ASO titer, history of scarlet fever, and a positive strep throat culture.

Jones Criteria:

Major Manifestations	Minor Manifestations
Polyarthritis	Fever
Carditis	Arthralgia
Chorea	History of RF or RHD
Erythema marginatum	Acute phase reactants (ESR, CRP)
Subcutaneous nodules	Prolonged P-R interval

d. **Medical Interventions**
  – **Medications** — Administer penicillin, erythromycin, sulfadiazine, anti-inflammatories (prednisone) and salicylates (to reduce the inflammation); begin prophylactic antibiotic therapy once inflammation is resolved; phenobarbital, chlorpromazine or diazepam may be used to treat chorea. Monthly injections of benzathine penicillin G or oral penicillin daily are given as prophylaxis
  – **Treatment** — Keep patient on bedrest to prevent stress and injury to the joints and heart
  – **Surgery** — Rheumatic mitral stenosis may be treated with percutaneous mitral balloon valvotomy; heart transplant for end stage cardiomyopathy

e. **Nursing Interventions**
  – **Assessment and Actions**
    * Be alert to signs and symptoms which may indicate rheumatic fever
    * Provide method of reducing discomfort (warm compresses, positioning, analgesics, antipyretics)
    * Assess for signs indicating potential complications, signs of congestive heart failure
  – **Teaching**
    * Assist family in understanding disease process and cause
    * Explain importance of keeping child on bedrest until disease is resolved
    * Encourage family to provide adequate nutrition to promote healing during active disease state
    * Emphasize importance of compliance with long-term prophylaxis and medication administration
    * Teach parents and child about medication prescribed (drug, dose, route, time and side effects)
  – **Emotional Care**
    * Promote growth and development
    * Provide support to family and child
    * Provide support group information to family

f. **Potential Complications** — Permanent cardiac damage to valves, death.

4. **KAWASAKI DISEASE**

a. **Description** — Kawasaki disease, or mucocutaneous lymph node syndrome, is an acute inflammatory disorder of unknown etiology. It involves many systems, most notably the heart. Eighty percent of the cases are seen in children under 4 years of age with a slightly higher male dominance.

b. **Signs and Symptoms** — Five of the six following criteria are required for the diagnosis:

1) **Fever:** Present longer than 5 days and not responsive to antibiotics

2) **Mucous membrane involvement:** Cracked, erythematous, fissured lips and a "strawberry tongue," oropharyngeal reddening

3) **Nonpurulent conjunctivitis:** Bilateral inflammation without exudate

4) **Polymorphous rash:** Typically involves trunk and extremities

5) **Lymphadenopathy**

6) **Digital swelling and desquamation:** Peripheral edema, erythema of the palms and soles with desquamation of the hands and feet

c. **Diagnostic Procedures** — The WBC, ESR, CRP, and platelet count will all be elevated; sterile pyuria and anemia may also occur. ECG shows prolonged PR interval; echocardiography may show pericardial effusion and is diagnostic for identifying coronary artery aneurysms or dilatation.

d. **Medical Interventions**
   - **Medications** — Salycilate therapy and intravenous gamma globulin (IVIG); anticoagulation therapy for children with large aneurysms
   - **Treatment** — Serial ECGs and echocardiograms to monitor coronary abnormalities
   - **Surgery** — Unnecessary

e. **Nursing Interventions**
   - **Assessment and Actions**
     * Monitor cardiac status, I&O, daily weight, rehydration
     * Be alert to signs and symptoms of CHF: decreased urinary output, gallop rhythm, respiratory distress, tachycardia
     * Administer medications on schedule and be alert to adverse reactions, salycilate toxicity
     * Provide symptomatic relief: mouth care and lubricating ointment to lips, skin care with unscented lotions, loose clothing, nutritional support with clear liquids, soft foods
     * Assess for signs indicating potential complications: change in cardiac status (cardiac monitor), signs of CHF, recurrent fever
   - **Teaching**
     * Discuss diagnosis and treatment plan with parents and child
     * Instruct parents and child on medication prescribed (drug, dose, route, time, and side effects)
     * Inform parents and child of signs of aspirin toxicity: tinnitus, headache, dizziness, confusion; low doses of aspirin may also cause easy bruising

- * Advise parents to notify the health care provider of any exposure to chickenpox or influenza due to the association of Reye's syndrome and aspirin
- * Administration of the influenza vaccine (yearly) and varicella vaccine is recommended
- * Teach parents the signs of cardiac ischemia and CPR
- * Avoid contact sports if long-term use of aspirin is required
- * Emphasize the possibility of a potential myocardial infarction
- * Instruct parents to provide a quiet environment and promote rest for the child and seek respite care for themselves as needed
  - **Emotional Care**
    - * Discuss impact of disease on child and family
    - * Provide support to family and child
    - * Provide support group information to family

f. **Potential Complications** — Coronary artery aneurysm, myocardial infarction, aspirin toxicity, allergic reaction to the gamma globulin, death.

5

GASTROINTESTINAL DISORDERS

I. General Concepts

- Gastrointestinal (GI) disorders may occur anywhere along the GI tract

- The GI system functions to provide nutrient ingestion, absorption, and elimination by mechanical and chemical breakdown

- At birth the GI system is immature and continues to grow in size and functioning ability until it reaches its mature size and functioning level during the schoolage years

- GI disorders may be congenital, acquired, acute or chronic

- GI disorders are one of the most frequently seen abnormalities in childhood and are frequently managed at home

- Dehydration from severe vomiting or diarrhea poses a serious threat and can occur rapidly

- Hospital discharge planning is important for the nurse to consider to enhance compliance with the treatment regimen and to maintain the child in a normal home environment

II. Specific Gastrointestinal Disorders

Congenital Disorders

1. CLEFT LIP/PALATE

a. **Description** — Malformation of the lip, maxilla, soft and/or hard palate. It may involve the lip and/or palate and may be unilateral or bilateral.

b. **Signs and Symptoms** — Lack of fusion of lip and/or soft or hard palate upon inspection.

c. **Diagnostic Procedures** — Diagnosed by characteristic physical findings.

d. **Medical Interventions**
   - **Medications** — Administer antibiotics postoperatively
   - **Treatments** — Based on defect; may also have increased frequency of otitis media which should be monitored
   - **Surgery**
     * *Cleft lip* — closure of lip(s) with sutures or reconstruction (when child is 1-2 months); sutures secured with Logan bow
     * *Cleft palate* — surgical closure after lip repair (when child is 4-18 months of age); may be done in stages

e. **Nursing Interventions**
   - **Assessment and Actions**
     * Assess newborn for defect
     * Provide adequate nutrition by using special nipples (Breck feeder, Lamb's nipple or special nurser)
     * Prevent aspiration by holding infant upright during feedings and aspirating excess mucus or formula from nose
     * Monitor hydration status and weight before discharged
     * Assist with organizing other healthcare professionals (speech therapy, audiology, nutritionist, occupational therapists, dentists)
     * Postoperatively — If lip repair: maintain Logan bow in place to reduce sutureline tension, apply elbow restraints; keep surgical area clean, observe for signs of infection, provide comfort measures, prevent vigorous sucking until lip area healed, some infants may breast feed, promote infant stimulation and interaction with parents; if palate repair: prevent any sharp object from going into mouth until area healed; restrain arms unless infant is attended by an adult
     * Assess for signs indicating potential complications
     * Administer pain medication

- **Teaching**
  * Explain defect, plan of treatment and time of typical surgical repair
  * Discuss potential need for dental prosthetic devices before and after surgery and necessity of good dental hygiene
  * Instruct parents on method of feeding, amount of formula, and length of time to allow infant to feed before and after surgery
  * Teach parent how to use bulb syringe if necessary
- **Emotional Care**
  * Facilitate bonding following birth
  * Determine parents' response to infant and provide support
  * Provide support to family
  * Provide support group information to family

f. **Potential Complications** — Minor physical deformity or scarring, chronic otitis media, speech deficits, difficulty in parents bonding with child.

2. CONGENITAL DIAPHRAGMATIC HERNIA

a. **Description** — The incomplete formation of the diaphragm during fetal development (most often resulting from the failure of the Foramen of Bochdalek to close) allowing the abdominal contents to herniate through a diaphragmatic hole into the pleural cavity. It most commonly occurs on the left side, and it requires emergency surgery. There is a high mortality rate if symptoms are present at birth.

b. **Signs and Symptoms** — Dyspnea, respiratory distress shortly after birth, flattened (scaphoid) abdominal appearance, vomiting, full or barrel chest appearance, difficulty feeding, absence of breath sounds on affected side of chest.

c. **Diagnostic Procedures** — Prenatal diagnosis is possible through the use of ultrasound. After birth, chest x-ray shows fluid and air-filled loops in the intestine in the affected side of the chest.

d. **Medical Interventions**
- **Medications** — Administer antibiotics, vasopressors, volume expanders, sedation, and pharmacologic paralyzing agents postoperatively
- **Treatments** — Maintain pulmonary function before and after surgery, do NOT face bag infant, prepare for intubation, place Salem sump to decompress GI tract, elevate head of bed to downward displace abdominal contents from chest, ECG and echocardiogram ordered to rule out cardiac involvement (hypoplastic left heart syndrome), extracorporeal membrane oxygenation (ECMO) immediately following delivery or during immediate postoperative period (these infants have a high mortality and morbidity rate related to persistent pulmonary hypertension)
- **Surgery** — Surgical repair of defect is essential and is performed immediately after diagnosis is made

e. **Nursing Interventions**
  - **Assessment and Actions**
    * Assess newborn for signs of defect
    * Preoperatively keep infant in high Fowler's position, place NG tube to prevent aspiration, administer oxygen as ordered, administer IV fluids, monitor for signs of severe respiratory distress
    * Postoperatively assess respiratory status, hydration status, bowel sounds, position infant in high Fowler's, administer sedations and other medications as ordered
    * Assess for signs indicating potential complications
  - **Teaching**
    * Explain defect, diagnostic procedures and treatment to parents, allowing time for questions
    * Inform parents of how infant will appear postoperatively
  - **Emotional Care**
    * Allow parents to interact and bond with child as soon as possible
    * Provide support to family

f. **Potential Complications** — Respiratory failure, circulatory problems before and after surgery, infection, Broncopulmonary Dysplasia (BPD — related to prolonged mechanical ventilation and persistent pulmonary hypertension), heart failure, death.

3. **IMPERFORATE ANUS**

   a. **Description** — An abnormality in the formation of the anorectal area. The malformation may be classified as low, intermediate or high anomaly. Other defects are often present.

   b. **Signs and Symptoms** — Depends upon location and type of defect: inability to pass stool, no visible anal opening, constipation and difficulty stooling, ribbon-like bowel movements, increased abdominal girth, inability or difficulty in taking rectal temperature.

   c. **Diagnostic Procedures** — Visual inspection, digital examination, and x-ray.

   d. **Medical Interventions**
     - **Medications** — Administer antibiotics postoperatively
     - **Treatments** — Depend upon location and severity of defect, but if mild includes digital or instrumental dilatation of anal opening
     - **Surgery** — Repair or reconstruction of anal opening or anastomosis of section of bowel not joined, placement of temporary or permanent colostomy may be required

   e. **Nursing Interventions**
     - **Assessment and Actions**
       * Be alert to signs and symptoms of disorder
       * Monitor stooling pattern before and after treatment/surgery

* Postoperatively monitor vital signs, surgical site, level of comfort, and provide method of pain control
* Assist with organizing home care service
* Assess for signs indicating potential complications

– **Teaching**

* Explain diagnosis to parents and discuss treatment regimen
* Teach parents how to digitally dilate area, if ordered
* Discuss with parents and child what to expect before and after surgery
* Teach parents colostomy and skin care prior to discharge, if needed
* Provide parents with anticipatory guidance and potential difficulty with toilet training if sphincter involved
* Teach bowel training regimen

– **Emotional Care**

* Provide support to family
* Provide support group information to family

  f. **Potential Complications** — Loss of bowel control, infection, perforation, permanent ostomy, skin breakdown.

4. OMPHALOCELE/GASTROSCHISIS

  a. **Description** — A malformation of the abdominal wall allowing intestinal contents to protrude either through the umbilical cord (omphalocele) or through the abdominal wall not involving the umbilical cord (gastroschisis). It is often associated with other anomalies.

  b. **Signs and Symptoms** — Visible defect at birth; abdominal contents protruding through abdominal wall.

  c. **Diagnostic Procedures** — Diagnosed upon inspection.

  d. **Medical Interventions**

– **Medications** — Administer broad spectrum antibiotics, sedation, parenteral nutrition, analgesics postoperatively

– **Treatments** — Maintain protective covering over sac preoperatively

– **Surgery** — Correct by returning abdominal contents to abdominal wall (either by gravity or surgical reduction)

  e. **Nursing Interventions**

– **Assessment and Actions**

* Be alert to signs of defect in newborn (defect may be detected on ultrasound prior to delivery)
* Postoperatively monitor vital signs, respiratory status, venous return, level of comfort; observe for signs of infection or rupture, assess bowel sounds

* Preoperatively maintain moist and sterile dressing on pouch, prevent rupture of sac, monitor vital signs, hydration, and temperature, position child supine, place NG tube and IV line
* Provide method for reducing discomfort
* Assess for signs indicating potential complications
  - Teaching
    * Explain defect to parents and treatment regimen, allowing for questions
    * Teach parents incision care and care of child at home
  - Emotional Care
    * Encourage bonding of parents with infant as soon as possible
    * Provide support to family

   f. **Potential Complications** — Rupture of sac prior to repair, infection, necrosis of bowel, obstruction, respiratory compromise postoperatively.

5. **PYLORIC STENOSIS**

   a. **Description** — The hypertrophy of the pyloric sphincter causing a narrowing of the normal passageway between the stomach and small intestines. It is most frequently congenital but may also be acquired and is seen in male infants more often.

   b. **Signs and Symptoms** — Projectile vomiting after feeding during second or third week of life; infant appears well and hungry but exhibits poor weight gain, distended abdomen with palpable olive-size mass in right upper quadrant, also exhibits visible peristaltic activity in abdomen, dehydration.

   c. **Diagnostic Procedures** — Diagnosed by characteristic history, physical inspection, ability to palpate olive-sized mass in right upper quadrant; x-ray after barium ingestion reveals stenosis (railroad track sign); ultrasound studies confirm pyloric mass.

   d. **Medical Interventions**
      - **Medications** — Administer antibiotics and analgesics postoperatively
      - **Treatments** — Place NG tube, correct dehydration and electrolyte imbalance
      - **Surgery** — Perform pyloromyotomy within 24 hours of diagnosis

   e. **Nursing Interventions**
      - **Assessment and Actions**
        * Be alert to signs and symptoms that indicate disorder
        * Preoperatively maintain hydration, fluid and electrolyte balance and keep infant NPO
        * Postoperatively monitor vital signs, hydration status, monitor bowel sounds and for signs of infection
        * Provide methods for reducing discomfort postoperatively

* Feedings start 4-6 hours postoperatively beginning with small, frequent amounts progressing to full feeding schedule in about 48 hours
- **Teaching**
  * Explain defect and treatment to parents
  * Discuss length of hospitalization (usually 3-4 days)
  * Teach care of incision
- **Emotional Care**
  * Continue to promote bonding between infant and parents
  * Provide support to parents

f. **Potential Complications** — Infection, fluid and electrolyte imbalance, dehydration, shock (prognosis is good).

6. **TRACHEOESOPHAGEAL FISTULA (TEF)**

   a. **Description** — A malformation of the esophagus and/or tracheal passageway. It may involve diversion of the esophageal contents into a blind sac, into the trachea, or into the trachea, then stomach or lungs. It can be life threatening.

   b. **Signs and Symptoms** — Difficulty feeding, coughing, choking; frequent regurgitation; becomes cyanotic during feedings; excessive drooling; typically has immediate onset of respiratory distress.

   c. **Diagnostic Procedures** — Diagnosed by inability to pass NG/OG catheter or by NG/OG tube curling back into mouth; fluoroscopic visualization of passing catheter shows obstruction or abnormal passageway; x-ray with radiopaque catheter shows dilated upper esophageal pouch.

   d. **Medical Interventions**
      - **Medications** — Administer antibiotics prophylactically and postoperatively; sedation and analgesics postoperatively
      - **Treatments** — Provide IV hydration and nutrition, prevent aspiration, place Salem sump tube to low intermittent suction, monitor for pulmonary infections
      - **Surgery** — Requires surgical dilatation, anastamosis of esophageal passageway with placement of temporary gastrostomy or cervical esophagostomy

   e. **Nursing Interventions**
      - **Assessment and Actions**
        * Be alert to signs and symptoms that indicate disorder
        * Preoperatively monitor vital signs, hydration status, respiratory function, keep NPO, prevent aspiration, keep infant comfortable, have suction equipment available, try to prevent excessive crying, keep head of bed elevated
        * Postoperatively monitor vital signs, hydration status, I&O, respiratory status, incision, observe for signs of infection or perforation

* Provide means for reducing discomfort
* Assess for signs indicating potential complications

   – **Teaching**

* Explain diagnosis to parents and explain treatment regimen
* Instruct parents on suctioning, feeding technique, signs of respiratory difficulty if treatment is delayed or to be done in stages
* Teach ostomy care and how to feed child through esophagostomy if surgical correction is to be performed
* Teach parents how to use bulb syringe

   – **Emotional Care**

* Encourage parents to care for infant to promote bonding
* Provide support to family
* Provide support group information to family

f. **Potential Complications** — Aspiration, pneumonia, dehydration, infection, esophageal strictures, death from aspiration or lack of patency of trachea to lungs.

Acquired Disorders

1. **APPENDICITIS (ACUTE)**

   a. **Description** — A swelling or inflammation of the appendix (vermiform appendix). It may lead to perforation and peritonitis if it is left untreated. It occurs more commonly in the school-age child.

   b. **Signs and Symptoms** — Fever, abdominal tenderness at McBurney's point, rebound tenderness in lower right abdomen, diminished bowel sounds, vomiting, legs drawn up to chest while lying down.

   c. **Diagnostic Procedures** — Elevated WBC present, x-ray reveals right curve of spine due to muscle spasm, fecalith may be visible. If perforation has occurred, free peritoneal fluid is visible on x-ray.

   d. **Medical Interventions**

     – **Medications** — Administer antibiotics postoperatively and preoperatively if rupture occurred, analgesics postoperatively

     – **Treatments** — Monitor I&O and discomfort pre and postoperatively

     – **Surgery** — Surgical removal (appendectomy) is necessary to prevent rupture and potential peritonitis; if rupture occurs, surgical correction must be performed immediately

   e. **Nursing Interventions**

     – **Assessment and Actions**

* Be alert to signs and symptoms that indicate disorder
* Preoperatively observe for signs of rupture: sudden absence of pain and change in vital signs indicating sepsis or shock
* Assess for level of comfort and provide method for reducing discomfort before, during and after surgery

* Postoperatively assess vital signs, bowel sounds, fluid and electrolyte status; position in semi-Fowler's or on right side, monitor for signs of infection
* Assess for signs indicating potential complications

– **Teaching**

* Explain procedures and surgical interventions to parents and child
* Discuss presence and purpose of postoperative equipment and treatment (penrose drain, NG tube, I.V. fluids, NPO status)
* Teach parents about medications prescribed (drug, dose, route, time, and side effects)

– **Emotional Care**

* Provide support to family and child
* Encourage parent to stay with child if possible

f. **Potential Complications** — Preoperatively, if rupture occurs, peritonitis, shock; postoperatively, infection.

2. **CELIAC DISEASE (GLUTEN-SENSITIVE ENTEROPATHY)**

a. **Description** — The inability of the bowel to tolerate gluten (protein found in oats, rye, barley and wheat). This intolerance causes problems with absorption of fats, carbohydrates, proteins, vitamins D, B12, and K, calcium, iron, and folic acid in the bowel. It is rarely seen in Blacks and Asians. Signs and symptoms typically appear before 2 years of age or after age 5.

b. **Signs and Symptoms** — Diarrhea, constipation, vomiting, abdominal tenderness and distension, anemia, failure to gain weight, irritability, apathy, loss of subcutaneous fat, muscle wasting, dependent edema in lower extremities; celiac crisis-bulky, greasy, frothy, pale, foul smelling stools (steatorrhea), smooth tongue, atrophy in extremities and buttocks, and edema.

c. **Diagnostic Procedures** — Stool analysis reveals steatorrhea, small bowel biopsy reveals alteration in villi, D-xylose absorption test and lactose H2 breath test are abnormal; sweat chloride test performed to rule out cystic fibrosis.

d. **Medical Interventions**

– **Medications** — Administer corticosteroid (prn), vitamin and mineral supplements, TPN if severely malnourished
– **Treatments** — Life-long dietary restriction of gluten-containing products (rye, oats, barley)
– **Surgery** — Unnecessary

e. **Nursing Interventions**

– **Assessment and Actions**

* Be alert for signs and symptoms
* Monitor child's growth and development
* Assess for signs indicating potential complications

- **Teaching**
  * Explain diagnosis and implications of treatment regimen to parents and child
  * Instruct parents on gluten-free diet (no ingestion of oats, wheat, rye, and barley) and importance of adherence throughout child's life
  * Teach parents and child causes of celiac crisis: poor diet adherence, stress, and infection; discuss potential life threatening nature of crisis (may cause dehydration and metabolic acidosis)
- **Emotional Care**
  * Provide support to family and child
  * Discuss how disease is impacting child and family's lifestyle
  * Provide support group information to family

f. **Potential Complications** — If diet not adhered to relapse may occur; long-term noncompliance may lead to anemia, growth retardation, osteomalacia, GI problems (change in mucosal lining, potential increase in incidence of cancer); celiac crisis.

3. **GASTROENTERITIS/DIARRHEA (ACUTE)**

   a. **Description** — An inflammation of the stomach and intestines which may be acute or chronic and causes diarrhea. It may be caused by a variety of organisms, nutritional intake, anatomical disturbance, allergies, disease processes, toxic ingestion, or neoplastic abnormalities. It is frequently seen in the pediatric population.

   b. **Signs and Symptoms** — Depend upon severity, causative factor, duration and age of child; presence of frequent diarrheal episodes, dehydration, fluid and electrolyte disturbances; may lead to shock if severe.

   c. **Diagnostic Procedures** — Diagnostic tests vary with causative factors; stool cultures determine if ova or parasites, blood, mucous, bacteria present; dietary intake assessment (determines if lactose intolerance present), x-rays check for obstruction or abnormality, blood cultures used to determine if organisms present; may also screen for toxic ingestion.

   d. **Medical Interventions**
      - **Medications** — Administer antibiotics (if caused by organisms), antispasmodics, or bismuth subsalicylate
      - **Treatments** — Discontinue foods and fluids containing lactose; mild and moderate dehydration may be treated at home by offering child oral glucose-electrolyte fluids (ex: Pedialyte); if dehydration is severe, IV fluids are necessary to achieve fluid and electrolyte balance; offer regular diet after rehydration
      - **Surgery** — Unnecessary unless mass or defect noted

   e. **Nursing Interventions**
      - **Assessment and Actions**
        * Be alert to signs and symptoms that indicate disorder

* Assist with determining level of dehydration (mild, moderate, severe) and causative factor
* Provide care according to severity of dehydration and cause:
  - **Mild and moderate** — Instruct parents on home care on increasing fluids, changing type of diet and/or medication therapy, and inform parents to call if signs of dehydration and diarrhea persist
  - **Severe** — Hospitalization required, monitor weight, I&O, vital signs, maintain IV site; monitor and record stools (frequency, consistency, amount, appearance), provide method for reducing discomfort and prevent perineal skin breakdown; isolation and enteric precautions may be necessary, depending upon the causative factor
* Provide progressive diet as ordered (liquids, to soft diet, to full diet)
* Assess for signs indicating potential complications
- **Teaching**
  * Explain diagnosis to parent and child
  * Instruct parent if child is to be cared for at home how to administer a progressive diet: liquids to soft to full diet or if dietary cause to remove source of irritant from child's diet
  * Teach parent how to prevent skin breakdown of the buttocks and perineal area and prevent secondary infections
  * Instruct parent to observe for signs of severe dehydration and when to notify the physician if symptoms worsen
- **Emotional Care**
  * Provide support to family and child
f. **Potential Complications** — Skin breakdown, metabolic acidosis, severe dehydration may cause shock and death if left untreated.

4. GASTROESOPHAGEAL REFLUX

a. **Description** — The presence of an abnormality in the cardiac sphincter allowing the stomach contents to flow back into the esophagus. It is frequently seen in infants (particularly preterm) until sphincter control is achieved.

b. **Signs and Symptoms** — Frequent, nonforceful vomiting especially after feedings, failure to thrive, esophagitis with bleeding noted in area, cyanosis, apnea, aspiration pneumonia, choking, and irritability.

c. **Diagnostic Procedures** — Diagnosed by characteristic history and physical; barium esophagram reveals reflux, esophageal manometry assesses motility and lower esophageal sphincter pressure, pH probe placed anterior to sphincter indicates higher pH in esophagus.

d. **Medical Interventions**
  - **Medications** — Administer bethanecol or metaclopromide, antacids, cimetidine (may be required)

- **Treatments** — If weight loss is not occurring in infancy, then treatment is unnecessary; if Failure to Thrive (FTT) or apparent weight loss present, encourage parent to feed child in upright position, include cereal in formula
- **Surgery** — Surgical correction may be necessary if severe reflux present (Nissen fundoplication)

e. **Nursing Interventions**
   - **Assessment and Actions**
     * Be alert to signs that indicate disorder
     * Monitor child's weight, I&O; measure amount, frequency, contents and time of vomiting
     * Maintain reflux precautions (place prone with elevated head of bed on slant board or with harness)
     * Provide method of reducing discomfort postoperatively
     * Assess for signs indicating potential complications
   - **Teaching**
     * Inform parents of diagnosis and treatment regimen
     * Teach parents how to feed infant: offer small amounts of fluid to infant with infant in an upright position, burp frequently, after feeding hold infant in upright position or place infant prone with head of bed elevated (30 degrees)
     * Teach parents about medications prescribed (drug, dose, route, time, and side effects)
     * Teach parents how to use a bulb syringe
   - **Emotional Care**
     * Prepare parents emotionally for child's surgery if required
     * Provide support to family

f. **Potential Complications** — Aspiration, anemia (if blood loss present), esophageal strictures, insufficient weight gain, apnea.

5. **HIRSCHSPRUNG DISEASE (CONGENITAL AGANGLIONIC MEGACOLON)**

   a. **Description** — A congenital abnormality in motility of a portion of the intestine causing an obstruction. It is due to an irregularity in innervation of bowel in which a segment is aganglionic and lacks peristalsis. The colon proximal to the defect enlarges due to lack of peristalsis in the affected area of the colon.

   b. **Signs and Symptoms** — Newborn's inability to pass meconium within first 24-48 hours, stool absent on rectal examination, increasing abdominal girth, bile-stained emesis, irritability, reluctance to feed, FTT, vomiting, constipation, explosive diarrhea. Childhood symptoms include abdominal firmness and distension, thin, foul-smelling ribbon-like bowel movements, constipation, poor weight gain.

c. **Diagnostic Procedures** — X-ray demonstrates dilated loops of intestine in absence of rectal air; barium enema reveals narrowed segment of bowel; rectal manometry reveals absence of relaxation of internal sphincter; rectal biopsy confirms diagnosis.

d. **Medical Interventions**
   - **Medications** — Administer antibiotics postoperatively
   - **Treatments** — Most children require surgery; enema therapy preoperatively
   - **Surgery** — Correct by removing defective bowel, may be accompanied by temporary colostomy placement, rarely removal of entire colon and placement of permanent ileostomy

e. **Nursing Interventions**
   - **Assessment and Actions**
     * Be alert to signs and symptoms indicating disorder
     * Monitor child's weight, I&O, fluid and electrolyte status, and abdominal girth
     * Postoperatively keep child NPO, assess vital signs and for signs of infection, maintain hydration and assess bowel sounds, observe for signs of peritonitis or perforation of bowel, provide method for reducing discomfort
     * Assist with establishing home care
     * Assess for signs indicating potential complications
   - **Teaching**
     * Explain disorder and treatment regimen to parents
     * If enema therapy is ordered instruct parents on how to administer, amount to instill, and importance of using normal saline solution
     * Teach parents how to care for colostomy, obtain return demonstration and discuss nutritional needs before discharge
   - **Emotional Care**
     * Promote growth and development
     * Provide support to family and child
     * Provide support group information to family

f. **Potential Complications** — Perforation and sepsis, peritonitis, poor bowel control, alteration in bonding, altered body image (child), persistent diarrhea, overflow incontinence, death.

6. **INFLAMMATORY BOWEL DISEASE**
   Ulcerative Colitis and Crohn's Disease*

a. **Descriptions**
   - **Ulcerative Colitis** — An inflammatory disease of the mucosa and submucosa of the colon and rectum. It is typically seen in young adults, but may affect any age. It is more common in Caucasians, upper socioeconomic classes and Jewish populations (a familial

tendency is suspected). It is a chronic disorder with unknown etiology.

– **Crohn's Disease** — Transmural inflammation of the intestinal tract wall. Affected areas repeatedly become inflamed and heal, causing scarring and weakening of the intestine. It may affect any area from the mouth to the anus but most commonly affects the terminal ileum and anus. It is also more common among Caucasians and the Jewish population with a familial tendency noted. There are often several areas of intestine affected at the same time. It is also known as regional enteritis.

Both typically occur in the late schoolage or early adolescence age group.

b. **Signs and Symptoms** — Signs and symptoms are similar and include anemia, fever, dehydration, fluid and electrolyte disturbances, stools containing blood and/or mucous, delay in sexual maturation.

COMPARISON OF SIGNS AND SYMPTOMS	
ULCERATIVE COLITIS	**CROHN'S DISEASE**
• Severe bloody diarrhea	• Frequent, watery diarrhea with or without blood
• Failure to thrive	• Abdominal pain (frequent)
• Abdominal pain	• Weight loss (severe)
• Weight loss (moderate)	• Moderate/severe anorexia
• Mild/moderate anorexia	• Severe growth failure
• Mild growth failure	• Rectal bleeding uncommon
• Rectal bleeding common	• Fissures/fistulas on barium enema
• Normal barium enema	

c. **Diagnostic Procedures** — (Both) stool analysis reveals blood and leukocytes; sigmoidoscopy reveals colitis; CBC may reveal anemia, leukocytosis, thrombocytosis, and increased ESR; barium enema reveals colitis; differentiated by intestinal biopsy; Ulcerative colitis reveals diffuse mucosal involvement with superficial ulcerations that are localized and contiguous; Crohn's disease reveals transmural lesions with deep ulcerations that are scattered throughout the intestine.

d. **Medical Interventions**

– **Medications** — Same for both disorders; administer sulfasalazine, corticosteroids, antispasmodics, immunosuppressive agents, and total parenteral nutrition

– **Treatments** — Provide nutrition; total parenteral nutrition may be used to allow bowel to rest during exacerbations

– **Surgery** — Surgical removal of affected bowel (colectomy) may be cure for ulcerative colitis; surgical resection for Crohn's disease is not beneficial due to the multiple patches present, surgical repair for complications of Crohn's disease may be needed and individual may need colostomy placement

e. **Nursing Interventions** — Same for both disorders
    − **Assessment and Actions**
       * Be alert to signs and symptoms
       * Postoperatively, monitor vital signs, abdominal girth, bowel sounds, suture line, and level of comfort
       * Provide method for reducing discomfort
       * Assess for signs indicating potential complications
    − **Teaching**
       * Explain diagnosis and treatment regimen to parent and child
       * Instruct parents and child about diet therapy — high protein, low fat, low fiber, high calorie diet
       * Inform parents and child of signs of exacerbations and remissions of disease and treatment required
       * Teach parents and child about medication prescribed (drug, dose, route, time, and side effects)
       * Discuss care of colostomy or ileostomy, if necessary
       * Emphasize need for follow-up care (increased incidence of colorectal cancer with each disorder)
    − **Emotional Care**
       * Promote child's body image and self-esteem
       * Encourage reducing stress as much as possible
       * Provide support to family and child
       * Provide support group information to family and child

f. **Potential Complications** — Same for both disorders: perforation and sepsis; peritonitis; skin breakdown around ostomy; medications and stress level increased leading to exacerbations; malabsorption; growth retardation; at higher risk for colon cancer.

7. **INTUSSUSCEPTION**

a. **Description** — A telescoping of a portion of the intestine into itself causing an obstruction. It is the most common cause of intestinal obstruction in the first 2 years of life. The etiology is unknown. It is more common in children with gastroenteritis, cystic fibrosis, and celiac disease.

b. **Signs and Symptoms** — Paroxysmal, episodic acute pain in the abdomen, vomiting, stools change from normal to a "currant jelly" appearance with red tinge; a long, cylindrical mass may be palpable in affected area; may be life threatening if bowel perforates or becomes necrotic.

c. **Diagnostic Procedures** — Diagnosed by physical findings, x-ray reveals area affected, barium enema reveals affected area.

d. **Medical Interventions**
   - **Medications** — Antibiotics may be given after reduction
   - **Treatments** — Hydrostatic reduction by barium enema; IV fluids
   - **Surgery** — If treatment is unsuccessful, then laparotomy and surgical reduction is necessary

e. **Nursing Interventions**
   - **Assessment and Actions**
     * Be alert to signs and symptoms
     * Assess for signs of rupture or necrosis prior to correction of defect
     * Postcorrection care includes monitoring vital signs, assessing and monitoring bowel sounds and stooling, maintaining hydration status, providing method for reducing discomfort, monitoring for signs of infection and shock
     * Assess for signs indicating potential complications
   - **Teaching**
     * Inform parents about diagnosis and treatment regimen
   - **Emotional Care**
     * Encourage parents to stay with child
     * Provide support to family and child

f. **Potential Complications** — Perforation, necrosis, peritonitis, recurrence of telescoping, death.

8. **VOMITING**

   a. **Description** — The expulsion of stomach or intestinal contents. It may be due to a variety of factors which include obstruction, infection, allergic reaction, toxins, tumors, and overfeeding.

   b. **Signs and Symptoms** — Expulsion of stomach or intestinal contents containing either liquid or food particles; may vary in color, amount, frequency, forcefulness, odor and duration.

   c. **Diagnostic Procedures** — X-ray determines if obstruction is present; review of history determines if vomiting is due to other medications, food, obstruction, infection, or possible exposure to poison.

   d. **Medical Interventions**
      - **Medications** — Administer antiemetic and IV fluids if dehydration is present
      - **Treatment** — Treat cause, maintain hydration, monitor nutritional status, discontinue solid foods, administer clear fluids for 12-24 hours then utilize BRATS diet (bananas, rice, applesauce, toast, and saltines) and later advance to solids as tolerated
      - **Surgery** — May be required if obstruction is the cause of disorder

e. **Nursing Interventions**
- **Assessment and Actions**
  * Obtain thorough history of emetic episodes to include duration, frequency, color, odor, precipitating factors, alleviating factors
  * Assess child's hydration status, vital signs, weight, level of consciousness, dietary intake
  * Prevent aspiration by positioning child laterally
  * If hospitalized, monitor vital signs, weight, hydration status, fluid and electrolytes; provide method of reducing discomfort, assess vomitus for blood, pH, and record amount, color and duration; maintain patent IV and advance diet as tolerated and ordered
  * Assess for signs indicating potential complications
- **Teaching**
  * Discuss diagnosis and treatment regimen with parents
  * Teach parents home management: diet progression from clear liquids to bland foods to full foods as tolerated; antiemetic administration; other treatments depending upon cause (antibiotics, identifying and removing stress or allergic sources)
- **Emotional Care**
  * Provide support to family and child

f. **Potential Complications** — Dehydration, fluid and electrolyte imbalance, shock.

6

GENITOURINARY DISORDERS

I. General Concepts

- The genitourinary system functions to regulate the body's fluid and electrolyte status and remove metabolic waste products and toxins from the body

- The kidneys and renal system of the infant are immature, resulting in inefficient regulation and concentration of solutes and waste products

- Infants are unable to concentrate urine until the age of one year, therefore frequent voiding occurs

- Bladder control and toilet training are not encouraged until sphincter control is achieved (usually after 2 years of age)

- Bladder capacity increases with age:
  Infants — 60 cc
  Toddlers — 285 - 400 cc
  Schoolage — 840 -1000 cc

- Disorders of the GU system cause fluid and electrolyte imbalances, inefficient clearance of medications, and build up of waste products in the body; treatment and correction of disorders must occur promptly if long-term complications and possibly death are to be prevented

II. Specific Genitourinary Disorders

Congenital Defects

1. AMBIGUOUS GENITALIA

  a. **Description** — The malformation and poor differentiation of external and/or internal sex organs.

  b. **Signs and Symptoms** — Ambiguous genitalia: the overdevelopment of female genitalia or underdevelopment of male genitalia. It is related to hormonal influences in utero, either maternal or fetal. It may be classified as female pseudohermaphroditism (masculinized female), male pseudohermaphroditism (incompletely masculinized male), or true hermaphroditism (very rare), in which the infant possesses both ovaries and testes (external genitalia may appear fully masculine to almost completely feminine).

  c. **Diagnostic Procedures** — Diagnosed by buccal smear, chromosomal analysis, gonadal biopsy to determine sex, surgical observation of internal organs (laparotomy).

  d. **Medical Interventions**
  - Medications — Administer appropriate sex hormones to assist with development of secondary sex characteristics
  - Treatments — Varies by cause and is managed by a physician; provide psychological support
  - Surgery — May include reconstruction of vagina or penis

  e. **Nursing Interventions**
  - **Assessment and Actions**
    * Be alert to signs and symptoms
    * Assess vital signs, I&O postoperatively
    * Provide a method for reducing discomfort
  - **Teaching**
    * Explain diagnosis to parents and long-term implications
    * Explain surgical reconstruction and timing
    * Teach parents about medication prescribed (drug, dose, route, time, and side effects); also explain the importance of not discontinuing the medication unless they discuss it with their physician
  - **Emotional Care**
    * Reassure parents that their child has a genetically identifiable gender and there is an explanation for this occurrence
    * Explain the testing procedures, the type of information they yield, and the length of time they take to complete
    * Provide a supportive environment to openly discuss how the parents will explain this issue to other family members and friends

  f. **Potential Complications** — Emotional stress for parents and child, malignant degeneration of organs.

2. CRYPTORCHIDISM

a. **Description** — The failure of one or both testes to descend into the scrotal sac, usually during the seventh to ninth month of gestation. Incidence more frequent in premature males (20%), occurs in 3% of well male children and resolves in 80% by one year of age. Must differentiate from anorchia (the complete absence of testes) or retractile testes which results from an overactive cremasteric reflex. The incidence of retractile testes decreases as the testes enlarge with age and the cremasteric reflex decreases. Frequently associated with inguinal hernias; also subject to torsion.

b. **Signs and Symptoms** — Empty scrotal sac on palpation, may be palpated in inguinal canal. Usually found at birth or soon after. Positive family history.

c. **Diagnostic Procedures** — Diagnosed through repeated manual examination of scrotal contents over the first two years of life. Though most testes typically descend by the age of one, spontaneous descent does not occur beyond the age of one year.

d. **Medical Interventions**
   - **Medications** — Administer antibiotics postoperatively as needed
   - **Surgery** — Surgical correction (orchiopexy) is usually performed by 18 months; the testis is surgically brought down into the scrotal sac and kept in position for several days by a traction device of the surgeon's choosing. If cryptorchidism persists into puberty, sterility may result. When the testis cannot be positioned correctly, it may need to be removed to diminish risk of later malignancy

e. **Nursing Interventions**
   - **Assessment and Actions**
      * Assess newborn and male children less than one year of age for scrotal content bilaterally
      * Postoperatively monitor vital signs, hydration, level of comfort (use bed cradle to prevent pressure on surgical area), observe for signs of infection
      * Provide method for reducing discomfort
   - **Teaching**
      * Discuss abnormality with parents and treatment regimen; reinforce the importance of follow-up after the procedure
   - **Emotional Care**
      * Discuss infertility of child with parents if appropriate
      * Provide support to family and child

f. **Potential Complications** — Infertility, long-term increased potential for neoplastic changes if testes are not replaced in sac or removed.

3. HYPOSPADIAS / EPISPADIAS

a. **Description** — The malformation of the external urethral opening of the penis. Hypospadias, in which the defect is along the ventral surface, occurs more frequently and seems to have a familial tendency.

When the defect is along the dorsal surface, it is called epispadias. Epispadias is much more rare and is commonly associated with exstrophy of the bladder. The defects may be small or severe.

b. **Signs and Symptoms** — Abnormal location of urethral opening of penis, usually on the shaft of the penis or near the glans. Occasionally a hypospadias may be located on the scrotum or perineum. Epispadias can occur in girls as well as boys; it may be hidden by the labia majora and recognized only by a cleft in the clitoris and a large urethral opening.

c. **Diagnostic Procedures** — Diagnosis by inspection.

d. **Medical Interventions**
   - **Medications** — Administer antibiotics, antispasmodics or analgesics as prescribed postoperatively
   - **Treatments** — Unnecessary
   - **Surgery** — Perform surgical repair of urethral opening before the patient is 18 months of age, most frequently when the patient is 13-15 months of age

e. **Nursing Interventions**
   - **Assessment and Actions**
     * Assess newborn male for any abnormality of urethral opening, observe for any alteration in voiding
     * Postoperatively monitor vital signs, hydration status, signs of infection; prevent tension or pulling of catheter, monitor urine output
     * Provide method for reducing pain
     * Assess for signs indicating potential pain
   - **Teaching**
     * Explain abnormality to parents and discuss treatment regimen
     * Postoperatively, discharge teaching should include care of stents or catheters and information about the use and administration of any medications prescribed
   - **Emotional Care**
     * Preoperatively, because of the child's developmental age, fears of mutilation must be addressed, as well as the parents' concerns about the child's future reproductive capabilities and dangers related to anesthesia
     * Postoperatively, provide support and information to the family and child

f. **Potential Complications** — Scarring, fistulas, abnormality in physical appearance and function, need for further reconstructive surgery.

4. VESICOURETERAL REFLUX

a. **Description** — The back flow of urine from the bladder into the ureters and often into the kidneys. It is due primarily to a congenital malformation in the bladder/ureter junction at the ureter implantation points. Reflux can also occur secondarily to obstruction, infection, or neurologic dysfunction. It may be graded according to the severity of reflux (Grade 1-5). Abnormalities may be unilateral or bilateral.

b. **Signs and Symptoms** — Persistent and repeated urinary tract infections are the most common indicator of reflux.

c. **Diagnostic Procedures** — Intravenous peylogram reveals defect, voiding cystourethrogram and/or cystoscopy allows for visualization of defect.

d. **Medical Interventions**
   - **Medications** — Administer antibiotics to prevent/treat infection
   - **Treatments** — Teach bladder-emptying exercise
   - **Surgery** — May require surgical correction of defect or obstruction

e. **Nursing Interventions**
   - **Assessment and Actions**
     * Be alert to signs and symptoms
     * Postoperatively monitor vital signs, I&O, comfort level, and for signs of infection
     * Assess for signs indicating potential complications
   - **Teaching**
     * Explain diagnosis to parents and child and discuss treatment regimen
     * Teach parents about medication prescribed (drug, dose, route, time, and side effects) and importance of maintaining compliance
     * Instruct parents on watching for the recurring UTI, encouraging child to increase fluid intake, establishing a voiding schedule, and completely emptying bladder
   - **Emotional Care**
     * Provide support to parents and child

f. **Potential Complications** — Renal disease.

Acquired Disorders

1. **ACUTE GLOMERULONEPHRITIS**

   a. **Description** — An inflammation of the renal glomeruli believed to be related to an autoimmune complex disease. It typically follows a Group A Beta hemolytic streptococcal infection (usually upper respiratory or skin). It is more commonly seen in children from 4-7 years of age.

   b. **Signs and Symptoms** — Symptoms appear approximately 10 days after streptococcal skin or respiratory infection and include acute onset of gross hematuria, edema, hypertension, anorexia, cola-colored and cloudy urine, irritability, headaches, proteinuria; if disease progresses, may develop oliguria, and generalized edema (anasarca).

c. **Diagnostic Procedures** — Diagnosed by urinalysis which reveals red cell casts, protein, elevated BUN and serum creatinine; blood studies reveal elevated ASLO titer and hemoconcentration.

d. **Medical Interventions**
   - **Medications** — Administer antihypertensives, diuretics and antibiotics as needed
   - **Treatments** — Prevent complications of renal disease, promote bedrest, may restrict dietary sodium; may require peritoneal dialysis
   - **Surgery** — Unnecessary

e. **Nursing Interventions**
   - **Assessment and Actions**
     * Be alert to signs and symptoms
     * Implement bedrest, nutritional monitoring, and prevention of secondary infection
     * Monitor vital signs, fluid and electrolytes, and weigh every day
     * Assess for signs of CNS involvement (headaches, dizziness, seizures), note urinary output and color
     * Provide skin care to prevent breakdown
     * Administer medications as ordered
     * Prevention of infection to prevent further strain on kidneys
     * Assess for signs indicating potential complications (change in urine output, abnormal cardiac or respiratory sounds, change in neurostates)
   - **Teaching**
     * Explain diagnosis to parents and child and allow time for questions
     * Explain normal progression of disease to parents and child: edematous stage followed by diuretic stage, and then, return to wellness
     * Teach parents importance of complying with diet therapy and what foods and/or fluids are restricted
     * Discuss with parents importance of follow-up visits
     * Teach parents about medications prescribed (drug, dose, route, time, and side effects)
     * Teach parents infection-prevention measures
   - **Emotional Care**
     * Provide support to family and child

f. **Potential Complications** — During acute phase (the first 4-10 days) may cause skin breakdown, encephalopathy, cardiac enlargement, pulmonary edema, and acute renal failure; may develop chronic renal disease.

2. ENURESIS

   a. **Description** — Involuntary urination in a child who is at the age to achieve bladder control (primary enuresis, which follows a familial pattern) or has achieved bladder control (secondary enuresis, which has been associated with emotional distress). It is usually functional, meaning it has no physical basis. It may occur at night during sleep (nocturnal enuresis) and may be due to organic or nonorganic factors (disease process, infection, familial tendency, or stress). It is more frequently seen in boys. Enuresis may occur as a developmental delay as children with enuresis are frequently delayed in the mastery of other developmental milestones. Diurnal enuresis in children over the age of five years is usually associated with an organic problem.

   b. **Signs and Symptoms** — Voiding involuntarily after the age of 4-5 years.

   c. **Diagnostic Procedures** — Diagnosed by determining cause; may perform the following tests: urinalysis, urine C&S, x-ray to rule out mass or obstruction, psychological review.

   d. **Medical Interventions**

     – **Medications** — May administer tricyclic antidepressants and anticholinergic medications, for short-term management when behavior modification fails; results are usually temporary at best with, sometimes, serious side effects; antibiotics if UTI is the cause

     – **Treatments** — Treat according to cause; may include conditioning techniques (alarm mattress), bladder training exercises, psychotherapy

     – **Surgery** — Surgical repair performed if due to obstruction or malformation in urinary tract

   e. **Nursing Interventions**

     – **Assessment and Actions**

       * Be alert for signs and symptoms

       * Assess for signs of child abuse or sexual abuse

       * Assist with identifying cause by obtaining thorough bladder history (age of toilet training and method, infections, frequency of voiding)

       * Assess for signs indicating potential complications

     – **Teaching**

       * Explain diagnosis and treatment regimen to parents

       * Encourage limiting fluids prior to bedtime, setting up a schedule for toileting, and teach bladder training exercises

       * Teach parents about medication prescribed (drug, dose, route, time, and side effects)

     – **Emotional Care**

       * Identify and discuss parents' and child's feelings about problem

* Assist in identifying stressors in child's life and offer ways to reduce stress
* Promote child's self-esteem and diminish guilty feelings
* Provide support to family and child; enuresis will eventually remit without treatment if not due to a physical cause

f. **Potential Complications** — Emotional stress, poor sense of self-esteem, social isolation, urinary tract infections if obstruction is the cause.

3. **NEPHROTIC SYNDROME**

a. **Description** — Damage to the glomerular structure of the kidneys causing proteinuria, hypoalbuminemia, hyperlipidemia, ascites, decreased urine output, and edema. In the approximately 90% of children with nephrosis, the cause is unknown. It usually follows a previous infection. It may be classified according to duration and kidney damage (minimal change nephrotic syndrome, secondary nephrotic syndrome, or congenital nephrotic syndrome). It is more commonly seen in children 2 - 3 years of age. The prognosis is good but the child may experience a relapse.

b. **Signs and Symptoms** — Edema of face, abdomen, extremities; increase in weight, perineal edema, diarrhea, scanty dark-colored urine, lethargy, fatigue, hematuria, azotemia, proteinuria, hypovolemia; may experience respiratory difficulty if ascites is extreme.

c. **Diagnostic Procedures** — Diagnosed by presence of proteinuria, hematuria, elevated BUN and ESR, decreased creatinine clearances, renal biopsy reveals disease process.

d. **Medical Interventions**

– **Medications** — Administer antibiotics specific to organism; long-term corticosteroid therapy, immunosuppressant therapy, diuretics, and cytoxan pulses (small doses of cytoxan given quickly with hydration pre and postadministration) may be utilized

– **Treatments** — Hospitalization may be necessary initially, promote rest, provide diet with minimal salt

– **Surgery** — Unnecessary unless renal biopsy (punch or wedge resection) is indicated

e. **Nursing Interventions**

– **Assessment and Actions**

* Be alert to signs and symptoms
* While hospitalized maintain bedrest , skin integrity, hydration status, monitor vital signs and weight, promote nutrition, monitor electrolyte levels, elevate edematous areas above level of heart, abdominal girth measurement
* Administer medications as ordered and observe for complications related to steroid therapy
* Maintain diet as ordered

* Anticipate diuretic phase within 1-3 weeks after symptoms appear
* Assess for signs indicating potential complications
* Maintain skin integrity (edematous areas are more prone to skin breakdown)

   – **Teaching**

* Explain diagnosis and discuss treatment regimen to family
* Emphasize importance of bedrest, good skin care and treatment regimen while at home
* Instruct parents on home monitoring of urine for albumin
* Teach parents about signs indicating potential complications

   – **Emotional Care**

* Foster normal development of child
* Provide support to family and child

  f. **Potential Complications** — Relapse, infections, skin breakdown, social isolation (if frequent relapses occur), chronic renal disease, shock (from electrolyte imbalance), death if untreated.

4. URINARY TRACT INFECTION (UTI)

  a. **Description** — An infection of the urinary tract (urethra, ureters, bladder, kidneys). It may be acute, chronic, recurrent, or develop into a more severe GU disorder if left undetected or untreated. Kidney involvement often results from an ascending infection. It occurs more frequently in females due to the shorter urethra.

  b. **Signs and Symptoms** — May be asymptomatic, particularly in chronic form; symptoms often age-dependent: *infants* - vomiting, diarrhea, FTT (Failure to Thrive), febrile episode, change in voiding habit and odor; *children* - dysuria, incontinence, increased frequency, enuresis, vomiting, fever, cloudy and strong-smelling urine, flank pain, urgency.

  c. **Diagnostic Procedures** — Diagnosed by positive urine culture and sensitivity (C&S) and x-ray (if obstruction or defect is present).

  d. **Medical Interventions**

   – **Medications** — Administer antibiotic therapy (sulfonamide, ampicillin, amoxicillin, sulfamethoxazole-trimethoprim, cefaclor)

   – **Treatments** — Increase fluid intake, monitor I&O

   – **Surgery** — Surgical correction of defect or obstruction is performed if present

  e. **Nursing Interventions**

   – **Assessment and Actions**

* Be alert to signs and symptoms
* Assess for signs of sexual abuse
* Obtain thorough history to assist in determining causative factor

- * Assess for signs indicating potential complications (altered urine output color or frequency)
- – **Teaching**
  - * Explain diagnosis and discuss treatment regimen with parents and child
  - * Teach parents about medications prescribed (drug, dose, route, time, and side effects) and importance of administering antibiotics for 10 days, or the time prescribed
  - * Teach parents to monitor for signs of recurrence and to promote rest
  - * Teach parents to avoid using bubble bath and harsh detergents
  - * Teach female patients to wipe from front to back to avoid contamination from stool organisms
  - * Teach sexually-active females to urinate before and after intercourse
- – **Emotional Care**
  - * Provide support to family and child

f. **Potential Complications** — May lead to renal disease and renal failure if it is recurrent or becomes chronic.

7

ENDOCRINE DISORDERS

I.   General Concepts

- The endocrine system is composed of chemical secretions (hormones) manufactured by specific cells in the body and target cells which receive the secretions through different modes of transport and respond accordingly

- It functions to regulate metabolism, growth, reproduction and sexual development, as well as, allows the body to maintain fluid and electrolyte balances and respond to stress

- Endocrine glands include adrenal glands, ovaries, pancreas, parathyroid gland, pituitary gland, testes, and thyroid gland

- Hormone secretion is based on a negative feedback loop throughout the body

- The endocrine system plays a vital role in the child's growth and development

- Disorders of the endocrine system may be due to a variety of factors and may be congenital or acquired; acute or chronic

- Disorders may cause hyper or hyposecretion of hormones

- Early detection and treatment of disorders can limit many of the long-term effects

- Discharge planning is vital to provide in order to assist the family and child with coping, compliance and appropriate home management

II. Specific Endocrine Disorders

Acquired Disorders

1. DIABETES MELLITUS

a. Description — The inability of the pancreas to secrete sufficient amounts of insulin. It may be due to genetic abnormality, autoimmune disorder, illness or diet. Type I Diabetes (IDDM — Insulin Dependent Diabetes Mellitus) is more common in children and young adults.

b. Signs and Symptoms — Polyuria, polyphagia, polydipsia, hyperglycemia, glycosuria (with or without ketonuria), weight loss, fatigue, irritability, enuresis.

c. Diagnostic Procedures — Diagnosed by detecting glycosuria, fasting blood glucose less than 120 mg/dL, normal or elevated serum insulin levels, elevated hemoglobin A_1c.

d. Medical Interventions
  – **Medications** — Administration of insulin; may require IV fluid resuscitation if in ketoacidosis
  – **Treatments** — Monitor blood and urine for glucose, protein and ketones; maintain diet following exchange list; encourage daily exercise regimen
  – **Surgery** — Unnecessary

e. Nursing Interventions
  – **Assessment and Actions**
    * Be alert to signs and symptoms
    * Monitor vital signs, blood and urine glucose, hydration status, level of consciousness, change in moods
    * Encourage participation by child in controlling illness:
      - Preschoolers should be able to help with cleansing site for injection
      - Schoolage children should be able to draw up and administer own insulin and monitor urine and blood with guidance
      - Adolescents should be able to select food and make decisions regarding insulin needs during illness, exercise, and stress
    * Discuss importance of compliance to treatment regimen, (problems tend to arise, especially in adolescence)
    * Assess for signs indicating potential complications
  – **Teaching**
    * Provide family and child with information about diagnosis and treatment regimen
    * Prepare family and child for discharge by teaching
      - Administration of insulin including type, amount, frequency, administration of injection, injection sites
      - Urine and blood monitoring and charting of these records

- Meal planning and how to use the exchange list
- How stress, illness, exercise, and growth affect insulin needs
- Signs of imbalance and how to treat
  - ° **Hypoglycemia** — Rapid onset of symptoms, serum glucose less than 60 mg/dL, shakiness, irritability, dizziness, sweating, headache, tachycardia, shallow respirations, hunger, paleness, may lead to coma and death
  - ° **Treatment** —administer simple sugar immediately (orange juice, sugar, honey, candy, Coke); if insulin reaction occurs, administer glucagon
  - ° **Hyperglycemia** — Gradual onset of symptoms, serum glucose less than 250 mg/d, weakness, drowsiness, lethargy, nausea, thirst, Kussmaul respirations, fruity breath, confusion, polyuria, dry skin and mucous membranes, weak and thready pulse, may lead to acidosis, coma and death
  - ° **Treatment** — administer regular insulin, increase fluids; if DKA is present, hospitalization may be necessary to return to fluid and electrolyte balance
- Importance of exercise and foot care
- Importance of avoiding injuries

- **Emotional Care**
  * Allow time for questions and concerns about diagnosis
  * Encourage parent to allow child as much independence as possible in treatment regimen
  * Promote self-care
  * Promote normal growth and development
  * Discuss with family and child concerns about disease process
  * Provide support to family and child
  * Provide support group information to family

f. **Potential Complications** — Neurological complications, vascular changes and poor wound healing, retinal and kidney damage, impotence, death.

2. HYPOPITUITARISM (GROWTH HORMONE HYPOSECRETION)

a. **Description** — A decrease in hormonal secretions from the pituitary gland. It is most commonly associated with a previous insult to the pituitary area (tumor, infection, radiation treatment).

b. **Signs and Symptoms** — Retarded linear growth with normal weight for age after first year of life; retaining youthful appearance; delay in appearance of permanent teeth, delayed sexual development, premature aging; if tumor-related — may exhibit signs of headache or visual disturbances.

c. **Diagnostic Procedures** — Diagnosed by assessing the family history for short stature, reviewing history of child's birth, reviewing child's growth (height and weight) from infancy, reviewing skeletal and skull x-ray to assess bone ossification and presence of masses; CT scan may be used to localize tumor or lesion; endocrine studies reveal decreased or absent growth hormone.

d. **Medical Interventions**
   - **Medications** — Administration of biosynthetic growth hormones as soon as detected
   - **Treatments** — Monitor response to medication
   - **Surgery** — Surgical removal or irradiation of tumor, if indicated

e. **Nursing Interventions**
   - **Assessment and Actions**
     * Assist with detection by plotting growth chart and sexual development
     * Continue to monitor growth once treatment is implemented
     * Assess for signs indicating potential complications
   - **Teaching**
     * Discuss diagnostic tests that may be required
     * Discuss diagnosis and long-term treatment regimen with child and family
     * Discuss need for daily injections with child and family
     * Discuss signs and symptoms of hypoglycemia and treatment
     * Inform that most children who are treated will eventually reach an adult height but puberty is often delayed by 1-2 years
   - **Emotional Care**
     * Encourage family to treat child at appropriate level for age even though they appear smaller
     * Promote positive self-esteem in child (especially adolescent age group)
     * Provide support to family and child

f. **Potential Complications** — Social isolation, emotional problems, delayed growth; if untreated, child will never attain normal size.

3. HYPOTHYROIDISM

a. **Description** — An abnormally low production of hormones from the thyroid gland. It may be congenital or acquired, acute or chronic. It affects 1 in 4 newborns and is often referred to as cretinism.

b. **Signs and Symptoms** — Newborn asymptomatic initially, if untreated: slow growth, irregular movements, brittle hair, dry, flaky skin, small forehead with eyes widely spread (infancy), cold skin, bradycardia, sleepiness, fatigue, constipation, nonpitting myxedema, large tongue, hoarse voice, may lead to mental retardation if undetected and untreated.

  c. **Diagnostic Procedures** - Diagnosed by finding decreased T_4 (thyroxine), elevated TSH levels, delayed epiphyseal development, decreased creatinine clearance; may use radioisotope of iodine to detect thyroid function.

  d. **Medical Interventions**
- **Medications** — Administration of thyroid hormone (Levothyroxine)
- **Treatments** — Monitor response to medication therapy
- **Surgery** — Unnecessary

  e. **Nursing Interventions**
- **Assessment and Actions**
  * Be alert to signs and symptoms
  * Refer parents for genetic counseling
  * Assess for signs indicating potential complications
  * Maintain accurate growth charts
  * Monitor for achievement of developmental milestones
- **Teaching**
  * Provide information to parents and child regarding disorder, treatment regimen and effects on child
  * Teach parents about medication prescribed (drug, dose, route, time, and side effects), need for compliance, and possible signs of overdose
  * Inform that child may appear "hyperactive" when compared to previous activity level
- **Emotional Care**
  * Provide support to family and child

  f. **Potential Complications** — If untreated: growth retardation, developmental delays, irreversible mental retardation.

4. **HYPERTHYROIDISM**

  a. **Description** — The oversecretion of thyroid hormone. It has an unknown etiology. It is more common in adolescence.

  b. **Signs and Symptoms** — Gradual onset of symptoms: increased hunger, weight loss, constant movement, nervousness, goiter (in some cases), sleeplessness, tachycardia, cardiomegaly, vomiting, diarrhea, warm and moist skin, intolerance to heat, exophthalmos, staring expression, weakness.

  c. **Diagnostic Procedures** — Diagnosed by presence of increased T_4 and T_3 levels, decreased TSH levels, mass may be palpable on thyroid gland, enlargement of gland on CT, increased uptake of ^{131}I (radioactive iodine isotope).

  d. **Medical Interventions**
- **Medications** — Administration of antithyroid medication (propylthiouracil), propranolol, iodide

- **Treatments** — Maintain diet with increased calories, carbohydrates and vitamins; rest; decrease stress in environment
- **Surgery** — Surgical removal of thyroid (thyroidectomy) may be
  necessary

e. **Nursing Interventions**
   - **Assessment and Actions**
     * Be alert to signs and symptoms
     * Observe for signs of thyrotoxicosis (thyroid storm): sudden
       vomiting, irritability, tachycardia, hypertension, and elevated
       temperature
   - **Teaching**
     * Explain diagnosis and treatment regimen to parents and child
     * Assist parents with providing for increased nutritional needs,
       and understanding problems of hyperthermia and possible be-
       havior problems
     * Teach parents about medications prescribed (drug, dose,
       route, time, and side effects)
   - **Emotional Care**
     * Provide support to family and child

f. **Potential Complications** — Thyroidtoxicosis (unusual in children):
   thyroid crisis. **Signs and symptoms**: restlessness, vomiting, diarrhea, tachycardia, hypertension, hyperthermia, may lead to coma
   and death if untreated; usually due to an illness or discontinuing antithyroid medication. **Treatment:** Administration of antithyroid medication and propranolol.

Congenital Disorder

1. **PHENYLKETONURIA (PKU)**

   a. **Description** — A genetic error of metabolism that occurs in 1 in
      15,000 births. It is carried by an autosomal recessive gene and 1 in
      50-100 people carry the gene. These children have absence of
      phenylalanine hydroxylase (a hepatic enzyme) which allows the con-
      version of phenylalanine to tyrosine. Abnormal byproducts accumu-
      late in the bloodstream and are excreted via urine and sweat. They
      may also accumulate in the CSF or body tissue. The level rises with
      protein ingestion and leads to neural damage and mental retardation.

   b. **Signs and Symptoms** — Undiagnosed infants present moderate
      to severe mental retardation due to degeneration of the brain and de-
      myelinization of the nerves. Urine has a musty odor; may have ec-
      zema or seborrhea, seizures, hyperactivity, bizarre personality, and
      behavior problems. Child is usually blonde, blue-eyed, and fair-
      skinned due to failure to produce melanin.

   c. **Diagnostic Procedures** — Newborn screening is the most effective
      method. Phenylalanine levels 12 mg/d, a serum tyrosine level 3
      mg/d, and phenylpyruvic acid and o-hydroxyphenylacetic acid in the
      urine are confirmation. Initial newborn screen may produce a false

negative, rescreening at 14-28 days may be suggested. Questionable results should be referred for phenylalanine challenge.

d. **Medical Interventions**
   - **Medications** — None
   - **Treatments** — Dietary treatment is used for control; diet consists of amino acid restricted diet maintained through adolescence. Infants are given a reduced phenylalanine formula (Lofenlac®)
   - **Surgery** — Unnecessary

e. **Nursing Interventions**
   - **Assessment and Actions**
     * Be alert to signs and symptoms of PKU
     * Assess nutritional, growth and developmental status
     * Work closely with multidisciplinary team following child to ensure communication
   - **Teaching**
     * Explain meaning of diagnosis and medical treatment plan including dietary restrictions
   - **Emotional Care**
     * Encourage parents to have genetic counseling
     * Provide support to child and family

f. **Potential Complications** — Mental retardation, hyperactivity and other behavioral problems, altered growth, failure to achieve developmental milestones/tasks.

MUSCULOSKELETAL DISORDERS

I. General Concepts

- The musculoskeletal system is made up of bones, joints, and muscles
- It functions to provide movement, heat production, posture, support, protection, mineral storage, and production of blood
- Muscle and skeletal tissue increase in size and density as the child ages
- The skeletal system continues to grow and develop until after puberty is completed, and the epiphysis of long bones closes
- The skeletal system heals more quickly in children than in adults
- The musculoskeletal system is affected by nutritional intake and by other disease processes; for example, parathyroid disorders, renal disease, malabsorption syndrome

II. Specific Treatments and Nursing Interventions

Cast

Utilized to immobilize extremity and promote alignment healing

- May be made of plaster or synthetic materials such as fiberglass
- Prepare child for procedure, and describe sensations that may be felt (cold, wet, heavy)

- Assist with comfort measures and with resetting extremity

- Provide warmth until cast is dried

- Handle wet cast with palms of hands to prevent indentations

- Elevate cast on pillows

- Assess cast for odor, drainage, pain, and maintain smooth edges; use petals if needed

- Discourage the sticking of objects into cast to scratch extremity

- Assess skin for infection, mechanical abrasion, breakdown

- Assess neurovascular status distal to cast (capillary refill, sensation, temperature, pulse, color)

- Discuss with child and family the limitations of wearing a cast

- Teach crutch walking or means of mobilization

- Promote safety while cast is in place

- Discuss length of time cast will be in place

- Before procedure, prepare child for removal of the cast and the appearance of extremity underneath the cast

- If spica cast is utilized, never move child by picking up by bar; promote safety, identify method of transportation/mobilization for child, keep perineum clean, maintain hydration and increase fiber in diet to prevent constipation

Fixation

Surgical placement of pins or wires to restore alignment and give support to extremity or affected bone

- May be internal or external pin placement

- Internal placement requires monitoring for signs of infection and providing comfort measures

- External placement requires pin site assessment and care and monitoring for discomfort and infection

- Describe procedure to parents and child and what area will look like after placement

- Discuss care of pins (as appropriate) and limitations fixation presents

- Identify a method of mobilization for child and teach crutch walking

- Provide safety measures for child

- Discuss length of time fixation will need to be utilized

Traction

Utilization of weights and pulleys, straps or pins to return bone or muscle to normal position; includes manual traction, skin traction and skeletal traction

- Prepare child and family for type of traction utilized

- Describe limitations traction presents (immobilization)

- Discuss length of time traction will be needed

- Promote normal growth and development for child and enhance socialization when possible

- Check function, alignment and position of traction and body part

- Monitor skin for signs of infection or ulcerations

- Assess circulation and neurological status to distal extremity

- Maintain proper body alignment and position in bed

- Maintain free hanging weights

- Promote comfort, nutrition and hydration (prevents constipation)

- Teach child how to use trapeze correctly

- Place nurse call light within reach

- Provide safe environment (side rails up)

- Assess for weakness, contractures in uninvolved joints and muscles

III. Specific Musculoskeletal Disorders

Congenital Disorders

1. **CLUBFOOT (TALIPES)**

    a. **Description** — A unilateral or bilateral congenital malposition of the foot or ankle. Cause unknown but may have familial tendency. Seen more often in males.

    b. **Signs and Symptoms** — Visual detection of incorrect positioning of the foot or ankle; foot or ankle cannot be manually positioned into normal alignment and is rigid.

    c. **Diagnostic Procedures** — Diagnosed by characteristic physical findings and inability to manually return foot/ankle into alignment.

    d. **Medical Interventions**

    - **Medications** — Administer antibiotics postoperatively
    - **Treatments** — Return foot to functioning position as soon as detected; mild forms may require daily ROM, massage, and placement of corrective shoes (Denis-Browne splints), some forms may require serial casting, corrective strapping
    - **Surgery** — More severe forms may require surgical correction

e. **Nursing Interventions** *(See previous section referring to casts)*
   – **Assessment and Actions**
      * Be alert to signs and symptoms indicating disorder
      * Assess child postoperatively for discomfort and provide method for reducing discomfort
      * Postoperatively, monitor vital signs and neurological, circulatory status of distal area
      * Assess for signs indicating potential complications
   – **Teaching**
      * Explain diagnosis and treatment regimen to family
      * Instruct family on care of the child: ROM, proper placement and care of the child in Denis-Browne splints (limitations of movement, care in turning or carrying, time of application)
      * If casting or strapping is required, instruct parents on care of casts/straps and affected area, frequency in which cast/straps will be changed, and signs or symptoms which require further medical assessment
      * If surgical correction is required prepare child and parents for what to expect
      * Prepare family for discharge and necessary home care of child with a cast
   – **Emotional Care**
      * Provide support to family and child
f. **Potential Complications** — Infection, foot deformity and scarring.

2. **CONGENITAL HIP DYSPLASIA**
   a. **Description** — The congenital displacement of the femoral head from the acetabulum. It may be categorized as: preluxation, subluxation, or dislocation. It is more commonly seen in females than in males. It may be a unilateral or bilateral defect.

   b. **Signs and Symptoms** — Unequal gluteal or thigh folds, discrepancy in leg length, diminished ability to abduct affected side, pain with diapering, positive click or popping with Ortolani and Barlow test; if undetected in infancy, may note leg length discrepancy in ambulating child as well as uneven gait (Trendelenburg gait), and lordosis.

   c. **Diagnostic Procedures** — Diagnosed by characteristic physical assessment findings and x-ray which shows defect. Ultrasound, CT scan, arthography are also useful.

   d. **Medical Interventions**
      – **Medications** — If surgically corrected, administer antibiotics postoperatively
      – **Treatments** — Maintain hip in flexion and abduction (Pavlik harness, Frejka pillow, casting, or skin traction)

- **Surgery** — Surgical reduction and reconstruction may be necessary if not treated early in life

e. **Nursing Interventions** *(See previous section referring to casts)*
   - **Assessment and Actions**
     * Be alert to signs and symptoms indicating disorder (treatment before 2 months of age has the highest success)
     * If surgical reduction required, postoperatively monitor vital signs, circulation to area, for signs of infection
     * Provide method for reducing discomfort
     * Assess for signs indicating potential complications
   - **Teaching**
     * Explain diagnosis and discuss treatment regimen with parents
     * Instruct parents on treatment regimen; teach how to care for child in harness or pillow device, encourage keeping skin and device dry and clean, monitoring for skin breakdown, discuss how to handle and care for child
     * Teach cast care and handling, if appropriate
     * Postoperatively, or after casting, teach means for mobilization
   - **Emotional Care**
     * Promote normal growth and development
     * Provide support to family and child

f. **Potential Complications** — If left untreated, may cause permanent change in femoral head or acetabulum, avascular necrosis; if surgical interventions necessary, may encounter infection.

3. **DUCHENNE'S MUSCULAR DYSTROPHY (PSEUDOHYPERTROPHIC MUSCULAR DYSTROPHY)**

   a. **Description** — A sex-linked, inherited condition that primarily affects males which involves a progressive muscle weakness and wasting. Symptoms usually appear by 2-6 years of age.

   b. **Signs and Symptoms** — Progressive muscle weakness beginning in spine, shoulders and hips, clumsiness, developmental delay or difficulty in gross motor activities, difficulty getting up from floor (Gower's sign), frequent falls, waddling gait, muscle atrophy, enlarged calf muscles; may later exhibit lordosis; muscle-wasting eventually affects all muscles of the body (including heart and respiratory system) death usually occurs by age 20 from heart failure or respiratory infection.

   c. **Diagnostic Procedures** — Diagnosed by detecting EMG myopathy, muscle biopsy reveals degeneration and variation in muscle size and increased amounts of connective tissue, serum enzyme tests reveal elevated CPK. ECG and CXR are done periodically to assess cardiac involvement.

d. **Medical Interventions**

 – **Medications** — Administer antibiotics to treat respiratory infections, digoxin and diuretics during cardiac failure, calcium supplements to minimize osteoporosis

 – **Treatments** — Prevent complications and maintain child at optimal functioning level, utilize PT, promote diet therapy, maintain pulmonary hygiene

 – **Surgery** — May be required to release contractures, may require tracheostomy

e. **Nursing Interventions**

 – **Assessment and Actions**

 * Be alert to signs and symptoms

 * Prepare child and parents for diagnostic testing

 * Encourage exercise (swimming is excellent) and promote rest periods

 * As disease progresses, provide care for patient on complete bedrest (skin care, ROM, pulmonary care)

 * Refer parents to genetic counseling

 * Assess for signs indicating potential complications

 – **Teaching**

 * Explain diagnosis and discuss treatment regimen with parents and child

 * Explain progression of disease

 * Teach child how to utilize and develop accessory breathing muscles (diaphragmatic breathing exercises) and utilize CPT as ordered

 * Teach parents and child ROM exercises, application of braces and positioning to prevent contractures

 * Teach parents to keep environment safe

 * Teach parents and child how to use wheelchair; do tracheostomy care, use rehabilitation services and assistive devices

 – **Emotional Care**

 * Assist parents with promoting child's independence

 * Promote growth and development, self-care, and socialization as much as possible

 * Provide support to family and child

 * Provide support group information to family

f. **Potential Complications** — Contractures, obesity, infections, atrophy, cardiac failure, osteoporosis.

4. OSTEOGENESIS IMPERFECTA

a. **Description** — An autosomal dominant (more frequent) or autosomal recessive disorder in which there is a defect in the connective tissues and bone causing disorganized bone structure and, therefore, brittle or fragile bones. It ranges in severity of bone fragility.

b. **Signs and Symptoms** — Depends upon severity and classification: frequent fractures, blue sclera, dentinogenesis, short stature, often exhibit several fractures or healed fractures on x-ray, may have hearing loss.

c. **Diagnostic Procedures** — Diagnosed by characteristic physical findings, reduced cortical thickness of shafts of long bones; elevated serum phosphatase levels, and decreased platelet aggregation; often must rule out physical abuse due to multiple fractures noted on x-ray.

d. **Medical Interventions**
   - **Medication** — Unnecessary
   - **Treatments** — Prevent complications and treat fractures
   - **Surgery** — May require pinning of fractures (intramedullary rods) to strengthen area and permit correct alignment

e. **Nursing Interventions**
   - **Assessment and Actions**
     * Assess child's level of comfort and provide method for reducing discomfort
     * Assess child's ROM
     * Assess limitations in ADLs
     * Provide safe environment for child during hospitalization
     * Refer parents for genetic counseling
     * Assess for signs indicating potential complications
   - **Teaching**
     * Discuss diagnosis with family and child
     * Discuss necessity for child's safety and importance of limiting contact sports
     * Discuss chronicity of disease and how child may become somewhat less fragile with age
     * Instruct child and family on how to apply and adapt to corrective devices that may be utilized: casts, braces, splints, hearing aids, glasses
     * Encourage gentle care of child during ADLs
     * Teach parent and child use of wheelchair as needed
     * Discourage immobility to decrease atrophy and likelihood of refracture
   - **Emotional Care**
     * Promote growth and development
     * Provide support to family and child

* Provide support group information to family

f. **Potential Complications** — Maligned bone healing causing deformity, hearing and/or vision loss, often confined to wheelchair as an adult; death if severe form of disease is acquired at birth.

Acquired Disorders

1. **FRACTURES**

   a. **Description** — A break in the bone. It may be classified according to tissue injury and includes simple or closed, compound, or comminuted. The fractures that occur commonly in children include bends, buckles, complete, and greenstick fractures. If the epiphyseal plate is injured, bone growth may be affected.

   b. **Signs and Symptoms** — Pain, swelling, decreased movement, numbness, tingling, deformity, ecchymosis

   c. **Diagnostic Procedures** — Diagnosed by physical findings and x-ray which reveals abnormality in bone; lab values may reveal elevated serum bilirubin, decreased hemoglobin and hematocrit; may have elevated creatine alkaline phosphate, SGOT, and LDH, and elevated WBC.

   d. **Medical Interventions**
      - **Medications** — Administer antibiotics to minimize infection; pain medications will depend on the severity of the injury
      - **Treatments** — Realign and immobilize (casting or traction) injured area
      - **Surgery** — Surgical correction may be necessary (open reduction) with or without pinning

   e. **Nursing Interventions** *(See previous section referring to casts, traction and fixation)*

      - **Assessment and Actions**
        * Be alert to signs and symptoms indicating disorder
        * Provide method for reducing discomfort: ice, elevation, immobilization, pain medication
        * Monitor for signs of infection
        * Assist with identifying how child will ambulate if leg is involved
        * Assess distal area for neurovascular functioning
        * Assess for signs indicating potential complications
      - **Teaching**
        * Explain diagnosis and discuss treatment regimen with parents and child
        * Prepare child for casting procedure and discuss length of time cast will be in place
        * If traction is necessary, prepare child and family and instruct on immobilization
        * Encourage diet high in protein and calcium

- **Emotional Care**
  * Promote growth and development
  * Provide support to family and child

f. **Potential Complications** — Fat embolism, infection, altered growth in extremity.

2. JUVENILE RHEUMATOID ARTHRITIS

a. **Description** — An inflammatory condition of the joints and connective tissue. It is chronic and usually occurs before puberty. It may involve one or more joints and cycles through remissions and exacerbations. Age of onset is between 2-5 years and 9-12 years of age. Females have a slightly higher incidence.

b. **Signs and Symptoms** — Nonmigratory swollen, tender joints that exhibit decrease in ROM (lasting 3 months or more); often the stiffness is worse in the morning (gelling); fever, erythematous rash, leukocytosis, iridocyclitis. The disease onset may be systemic, pauciarticular (less than 5 joints) or polyarticular.

c. **Diagnostic Procedures** — Diagnosed by characteristic physical findings and history of persistent symptoms for three months; x-ray reveals soft tissue swelling and regional osteoporosis; often necessary to rule out other disease processes (cancer, rheumatic fever, Lyme's disease)

d. **Medical Interventions**
  - **Medications** — Administration of nonsteroidal anti-inflammatory drugs (NSAIDs, naproxen, tolmetin sodium, ibuprofen), slower acting antirheumatic drugs (antimalarials, gold compound, D-penicillamine, sulfasalazine), corticosteroids, cytotoxic medications, aspirin
  - **Treatments** — Maintain ROM and comfort, splinting and positioning to reduce flexion deformity
  - **Surgery** — May require synovectomy, joint replacement or joint fusion

e. **Nursing Interventions**
  - **Assessment and Actions**
    * Assess limitations in ROM
    * Assess for activities that cause exacerbations
    * Provide method for reducing discomfort: pain management, positioning, splinting, weight control
    * Assess for signs indicating potential complications
  - **Teaching**
    * Discuss diagnosis and chronicity with parents and child
    * Instruct parents on home therapy, ROM exercises (passive ROM after inflammatory period), splinting of affected extremities, application of heat, use of assistive devices such as tongs, self-adhering fasteners, grab bars

* Instruct on methods for reducing discomfort
* Encourage rest, well-balanced diet
* Encourage application of warm compresses or warm paraffin or whirlpool therapy to joints
* Teach parents about medication prescribed (drug, dose, route, time, and side effects), NSAID and aspirin toxicity
  - **Emotional Care**
    * Promote growth and development and self-esteem of child
    * Provide support group information to family

  f. **Potential Complications** — Contractures, cataracts, loss of joint mobility, severe hip disease.

3. **LEGG-CALVE-PERTHES DISEASE**
   a. **Description** — A self-limiting disease in which localized ischemia causes avascular necrosis of the femoral head. It results in degeneration of the femoral head and may affect the growth plate. It progresses through four states: avascular stage, revascularization stage, reparative stage, and regenerative stage. It is most commonly seen during 4-8 years of age with a male/female ratio of 5:1. It is often referred to as Coxa Plana or osteochondritis deformans juveniles. Ten percent of the cases are bilateral.

   b. **Signs and Symptoms** — May initially exhibit a limp, complain of soreness and pain in the hip joint, groin, thigh or knee, and display guarding or limitation in ROM. Pain is aggravated by activity and relieved by rest.

   c. **Diagnostic Procedures** — Diagnosed by evidence of deterioration of the femoral head by x-ray.

   d. **Medical Interventions**
      - **Medications** — Unnecessary
      - **Treatments** — Focuses on preservation of the joint and extremity throughout course of disease (may require 2 years of treatment), maintaining joint in acetabulum, placement of casts or braces to hold joint in abduction and internal rotation
      - **Surgery** — Surgical correction returns the child to normal activities within 4-6 weeks and may be preferable to the 2 years of casting and braces. Surgical joint replacement may be required later in life in 50% of the cases

   e. **Nursing Interventions**
      - **Assessment and Actions**
        * Assess level of discomfort
        * Limit ROM of affected extremity
        * Assess skin for areas of breakdown due to brace
        * Provide method for reducing discomfort
        * Assess for signs indicating complications

- Teaching
  * Discuss diagnosis with family and child and long-term treatment requirements
  * Instruct parents and child on importance of bedrest and compliance with treatment regimen
  * Instruct on proper brace application and discourage weight-bearing on affected extremity
  * Teach crutch walking or identify mode for movement
  * If bedrest and traction are necessary discuss with parent and child
  * Prepare parents and child for discharge and home care
- Emotional Care
  * Promote growth and development
  * Provide support to family and child

f. **Potential Complications** — Loss of ROM, growth disturbance in affected limb.

4. OSTEOMYELITIS

a. **Description** — An infection of the bone tissue usually preceded by an infection or injury somewhere in the body. It usually affects the long bones and may be an acute or chronic disease. It can occur at any age but is frequently seen in children under one year and between five and fourteen years of age. It is more common in males.

b. **Signs and Symptoms** — Pain in affected area accompanied by guarding, swelling, warmth over area, fever, irritability, diarrhea.

c. **Diagnostic Procedures** — Diagnosed by presence of a positive blood culture, periosteal culture, bone aspiration; an increased ESR, presence of leukocytosis, x-ray reveals localized swelling (periosteal culture, bone aspiration).

d. **Medical Interventions**
   - **Medications** — Long-term antibiotic therapy (organism specified), pain medications
   - **Treatments** — Maintain bedrest, splint affected extremity, physical therapy when infection subsides
   - **Surgery** — Surgical drainage of area or aspiration of fluid may be required; sequestrectomy, irrigation and debridement may also be required

e. **Nursing Interventions**
   - **Assessment and Actions**
     * Monitor VS, hydration status, and level of comfort
     * Maintain patent IV and administer antibiotics as scheduled (may be treated at home)
     * After treatment progresses and bone is infection free, slowly introduce ROM to extremity

* Provide method for reducing discomfort
* Assess for signs indicating potential complications
- **Teaching**
  * Discuss diagnosis and necessity for long-term antibiotic therapy (4-6 weeks)
  * Discuss with child and parents: limitations, bedrest, immobilization of extremity, avoidance of weight-bearing or use of affected extremity
- **Emotional Care**
  * Promote growth and development and socialization
  * Provide support to family and child

f. **Potential Complications** — Spread of infection to other sites, injury to bone, permanent loss of bone structure, growth abnormality of extremity.

5. **SLIPPED FEMORAL CAPITAL EPIPHYSIS (EPIPHYSIOLYSIS)**

   a. **Description** — The displacement of the femoral head from the neck of the femur. It is caused by a shift in the epiphyseal plate. It typically occurs during a growth spurt and is more frequently seen in obese adolescents. It may occur unilaterally or bilaterally and can be an acute or chronic disorder. It may or may not be preceded by a traumatic injury to the area and is seen more frequently in males.

   b. **Signs and Symptoms** — Intermittent or constant hip, groin or knee pain with decreased internal rotation of hip, decreased ROM of hip, and limping.

   c. **Diagnostic Procedures** — Diagnosed by physical findings and by visualizing displacement of femoral head on x-ray.

   d. **Medical Interventions**
      - **Medications** — Unnecessary
      - **Treatments** — Protect the joint and growth plate by stabilization and immobilization until surgical intervention
      - **Surgery** — Requires internal fixation with pins, skeletal traction, osteotomy, or open bone graft; epiphysiodesis for severe chronic slipped epiphyses

   e. **Nursing Interventions**
      - **Assessment and Actions**
        * Be alert to signs and symptoms
        * Provide method for reducing discomfort
        * Assess for signs indicating potential complications
      - **Teaching**
        * Discuss diagnosis with parents and child
        * Explain limitations of disorder: no weight-bearing on extremity, bedrest and traction
        * Teach child crutch walking and about traction

- **Emotional Care**
  * Promote growth, development and self-esteem
  * Provide support to family and child

f. **Potential Complications** — Altered growth in affected extremity, chronic pain or limping, avascular and cartilaginous necrosis of area, loss of ROM.

6. SCOLIOSIS

a. **Description** — The lateral curvature or rotation of the spine. It may be a structural (progressive disorder requiring mechanical or surgical correction) or a nonstructural (nonprogressive and voluntarily correctable, often due to poor posture) disorder. It can be congenital or acquired and varies in age of onset depending on the type. Most frequent is idiopathic scoliosis which has a female predominance and is most commonly seen during the preputeral growth spurt.

b. **Signs and Symptoms** — Visual malalignment of the spine, sternum is not in midline, visible unilateral hump noted on posterior along spine when child bends forward, hips/shoulders are not bilaterally even in height; poorly fitting clothes, especially swimsuits, bras, uneven pant legs or skirt hems; often asymptomatic.

c. **Diagnostic Procedures** — Diagnosed by physical findings and confirmed by visible malalignment on x-ray, scoliometer used for screening. MRI may be needed to rule out other disease processes.

d. **Medical Interventions**
  - **Medications** — Administer antibiotic postoperatively
  - **Treatments** — Treatment depends upon type, severity and location of disorder: nonstructural scoliosis — exercises to improve muscle strength and posture, utilization of external brace; structural scoliosis — exercises, brace, electrical stimulation
  - **Surgery** — Structural scoliosis may require surgical correction (spinal fusion, Harrington, Dwyer, or Luque instrumentation)

e. **Nursing Interventions**
  - **Assessment and Actions**
    * Provide screening to all teenagers, especially females, during physical examinations
    * Prepare child for wearing brace; describe fitting, hygiene, and when it can be removed
    * If surgery required, prepare child for surgical procedure and what to expect postoperatively
    * Postoperatively monitor child's VS, neuro and circulatory status, comfort level, hydration, nutrition, urinary elimination, constipation, and skin for signs of breakdown or infection; turn child by log-rolling and keep positioned in alignment
    * Assess for signs indicating potential complications

- **Teaching**
  * Explain diagnosis to parent and child
  * Explain treatment regimen and importance of compliance
  * Teach child exercise regimen and obtain return demonstration
  * Postoperative discharge education should include instructing child not to sit for long periods of time, to refrain from bending (squat instead), and to participate in only low-impact activities
  * Teach importance of safety for child in brace
  * Prepare child and family for discharge and home care, including how to perform physical therapy; modify diet to prevent overeating and constipation and provide adequate nutrition
- **Emotional Care**
  * Assist child in identifying clothing that will conceal brace
  * Discuss child's feelings of having to wear brace
  * Promote child's self-esteem and development
  * Provide support to family and child
  * Provide support group information to family

f. **Potential Complications** — Permanent skeletal deformity.

9

COMMUNICABLE DISEASES

I.　General Concepts

- Communicable diseases are caused by those infectious agents which are passed or transmitted via animate or inanimate objects (reservoir) to a host and which cause illness of that host

- Transmission may be through direct or indirect contact with infected item

- Children are more susceptible to communicable diseases due to the immaturity in their immune system and their increased interaction with the environment

- Communicable diseases require the nurse to attempt to prevent the occurrence, identify the disease quickly, provide treatment, prevent the spread, and prevent any possible complications

- Many communicable diseases may also be prevented by proper handwashing and hygiene, and limited exposure to infected children and objects that infected chidren have played with while in the contagious stage of the disease

- Many communicable diseases can be prevented by immunizing the child

- Occurrences of vaccine-preventable diseases (polio, pertussis, rubella, diphtheria, etc.) are reportable to state health departments

- Health care providers are required by law to report adverse effects experienced by the child after immunization

II. Prevention of Communicable Diseases

Immunizations

1. The following immunization schedule should be followed:

Recommended Childhood Immunization Schedule United States, January - December 1997

Vaccines[1] are listed under the routinely recommended ages. Bars indicate range of acceptable ages for vaccination. Shaded Bars indicate *catch-up vaccination*; at 11-12 years of age, hepatitis B vaccine should be administered to children not previously vaccinated, and Varicella vaccine should be administered to children not previously vaccinated who lack a reliable history of chickenpox.

Age → Vaccine	Birth	1 mo	2 mos	4 mos	6 mos	12 mos	15 mos	18 mos	4- yrs	11-12 yrs	14-16 yrs
Hepatitis B[2,3]	Hep B-1										
			Hep B-2			Hep B-3				Hep B[3]	
DTP[4]			DTaP or DTP	DTaP or DTP	DTaP or DTP		DTaP or DTP[4]		DTaP or DTP	Td	
H. Influenae type b[5]			Hib	Hib	Hib[5]	Hib[5]					
Polio[6]			Polio[6]	Polio		Polio[6]			Polio		
Measles, Mumps, Rubella[7]						MMR				MMR[7] or MMR[7]	
Varicella[8]						Var				Var[8]	

Approved by the Advisory Committee on Immunization Practice (ACIP), the American Academy of Pediatrics (AAP), and the American Academy of Family Physicians (AAFP).

DTP: Diphtheria, Tetanus, and Pertussis Vaccine
Polio: Live Oral Polio Vaccine drops (OPV)
or Killed (Inactivated) Polio Vaccine shots (IPV)

MMR: Measles, Mumps, and Rubella Vaccine
HIB: Haemophilus b Conjugate Vaccine
HB: Hepatitis B Vaccine

1   The schedule indicates the recommended age for routine admission of currently licensed childhood vaccines. Some combination vaccines are available and may be used whenever administration of all components of the vaccine is indicated. Providers should consult the manufacturers' package inserts for detailed recommendations.

2   Infants born to HBsAg-negative mothers should receive 2.5 µg of Merck vaccine (Recombivax HB) or 10 µg of SmithKline Beecham (SB) vaccine (Engerix-B). The 2nd dose should be administered ≥1 mos after the first dose.

    Infants born to HBsAg-positive mothers should receive 0.5 mL hepatitis B immune globulin (HBIG) within 12 hrs of birth, and either 5 µg of Merck vaccine (Recombivax HB) or 10 µg of SB vaccine (Engerix-B) at a separate site. The 2nd dose is recommended at 1-2 mos of age and the 3rd dose at 6 mos of age.

    Infants born to mothers whose HBsAg status is unknown should receive either 5 µg of Merck vaccine (Recombivax HB) or 10 µg of SB vaccine (Engerix-B) within 12 hrs of birth. The second dose of vaccine is recommended at 1 mo of age and the third dose at 6 mos of age. Blood should be drawn at the time of delivery to determine the mother's HBsAg status; if it is positive, the infant should receive HBIG as soon as possible (no later than 1 wk of age). The dosage and timing of subsequent vaccine doses should be based upon the mother's HBsAg status.

3   Children and adolescents who have not been vaccinated against hepatitis B in infancy may begin the series during any childhood visit. Those who have not previously received 3 doses of hepatitis B vaccine should initiate or complete the series during the 11-12 year-old visit. The second dose should be

administered at least 1 mo after the first dose, and the third dose should be administered at least 4 mos after the first dose and at least 2 mos after the second dose.

4   DTaP (diphtheria and tetanus toxoids and acellular pertussis vaccine) is the preferred vaccine for all doses in the vaccination series, including completion of the series in children who have received ≥1 dose of whole-cell DTP vaccine. Whole-cell DTP is an acceptable alternative to DTaP. The fourth dose (DTaP or DTP) may be administered as early as 12 mos of age, provided 6 mos have elapsed since the third dose, and if the child is considered unlikely to return at 15-18 mos of age. Td (tetanus and diphtheria toxoids, absorbed, for adult use) is recommended at 11-12 yrs of age if at least 5 years have elapsed since the last dose of DTP, DTaP or DT. Subsequent routine Td boosters are recommended every 10 years.

5   Three H. influenzae type b (Hib) conjugate vaccines are licensed for infant use. If PRP-OMP (Pedvax-HIB [Merck]) is administered at 2 and 4 mos of age, a dose at 6 mos is not required. After completing the primary series, any Hib conjugate vaccine may be used as a booster.

6   Two poliovirus vaccines are currently licensed in the USA: inactivated poliovirus vaccine (IPV) and oral poliovirus vaccine (OPV). The following schedules are acceptable by the ACIP, the AAP, and the AAFP, and parents and providers may choose among them:

    1. IPV at 2 and 4 mos; OPV at 12-18 mos and 4-6 yr
    2. IPV at 2, 4, 12-18 mos, and 4-6 yr
    3. OPV at 2, 4, 6-18 mos, and 4-6 yr

The ACIP routinely recommends schedule 1. IPV is the only poliovirus vaccine recommended for immunocompromised persons and their household contacts.

7   The 2nd dose of MMR is routinely recommended at 4-6 yrs of age or at 11-12 yrs of age, but may be administered during any visit, provided at least 1 month has elapsed since receipt of the 1st dose and that both doses are administered at or after 12 mos of age.

8   Susceptible children may receive Varicella vaccine (Var) at any visit after the first birthday, and those who lack a reliable history of chickenpox should be immunized during the 11-12 year-old visit. Children ≥13 years of age should receive 2 doses, at least 1 mo apart.

Source: Committee on Infectious Diseases, American Academy of Pediatrics (1997). <u>1997 Red Book: Report of the Committee on Infectious Diseases</u>. Elk Grove, IL: American Academy of Pediatrics.

2. Parents must sign a consent form prior to immunization administration.

3. Child should be screened prior to administration to ensure:

    a. Immunizations are up to date

    b. Previous reactions not experienced

    c. Child is not severely ill or does not have chronic illness

    d. No previous history of seizures or neurological disorders; if child's history causes concern, consult a physician

    e. Child has no allergies to ingredients in vaccines (e.g., neomycin)

4. Susceptible post-menarche females should not be vaccinated with live vaccines until counseled about the potential hazard to the fetus; also, counseled to use appropriate contraception to prevent pregnancy for three months after receiving live vaccines (e.g., MMR, OPV).

5. Make parents and child aware of normal and abnormal side effects and when to seek further assistance for child if reaction occurs.

6. Children with depressed immune systems should not receive active immunization with live vaccines. Inactivated vaccines and immunoglobulins should be used as needed.

7. Minor acute illnesses and fever of less than 38°C are not a contraindication for vaccination; however, a child with a moderate to severe illness with or without fever, or a child with a fever greater than 38°C,

should be assessed by the health care provider to evaluate the risks versus the benefits of immunization at that time.

Types of Immunity

1. **ARTIFICIALLY ACQUIRED IMMUNITY**
   Host is exposed to infectious organism artificially introduced into the host's body. Host then builds antibodies against future organism contamination. Duration of immunity varies and booster immunizations may be required (e.g., tetanus vaccination).

2. **ARTIFICIALLY ACQUIRED PASSIVE IMMUNITY**
   Host is injected with antibodies to specific infectious agent. Duration of immunity varies from weeks to months (e.g., gamma globulin, hepatitis B immune globulin).

3. **NATURALLY ACQUIRED ACTIVE IMMUNITY**
   Host is directly exposed to organism in external environment and builds antibodies after infected. Duration of immunity lasts throughout life (e.g., rubeola).

4. **NATURALLY ACQUIRED PASSIVE IMMUNITY**
   Host is exposed to antibodies through placenta while still in utero or through breast milk, protection lasts first 3-4 months of life.

III. Pediatric Communicable Diseases

Bacterial Infections

1. **Diphtheria**

   a. **Agent** — *Cornybacterium diphtheriae.*

   b. **At Risk** — Anyone who has not been immunized — highest incidence in children under 15 years.

   c. **Incubation** — Uncertain, but believed to be 2-5 days.

   d. **Communicable Period** — Variable, usually 2 weeks after symptoms appear but can be as long as several months.

   e. **Seasonal Incidence** — Common in fall and winter.

   f. **Transmission** — Direct contact by sneezing, coughing, and talking with infected person.

   g. **Diagnostic Procedures** — Positive nasal and throat cultures.

   h. **Signs and Symptoms** — Sore throat, visible membrane formation in nasopharynx area; may affect the nasal, tonsillar, pharyngeal, or laryngeal areas; malaise, anorexia, low-grade fever, lymphadenopathy, hoarseness, cough.

   i. **Medical Interventions**
       – **Medications** — Equine antitoxin IV (check for sensitivity to horse serum); erythromycin, penicillin G
       – **Treatment** — Palliative

- **Surgery** — Tracheostomy if airway obstruction

j. **Nursing Interventions** — Strict isolation, medication as prescribed, complete bedrest, observe respiratory status, high carbohydrate diet, increased fluid intake, obtain nasal and tonsil cultures — two serial negative cultures needed before isolation discontinued.

k. **Potential Complications** — Approximately 50% of children infected also develop myocardial complications and congestive heart failure, also may have temporary neuritis and soft palate paralysis, airway obstruction.

2. **PERTUSSIS (WHOOPING COUGH)**

a. **Agent** — *Bordetella pertussis.*

b. **At Risk** — Less common in immunized children, may affect infants and children — adolescents and adults account for 25% of the cases; can affect health care providers; can occur at any age.

c. **Incubation** — 5-21 days.

d. **Communicable Period** — One week prior and 3-4 weeks after symptoms appear.

e. **Seasonal Incidence** — Spring and summer.

f. **Transmission** — Droplets or contact with contaminated inanimate objects.

g. **Signs and Symptoms** — Upper respiratory infection signs and symptoms: low-grade fever; paroxysmal coughing worsens and is most frequent at night, often sounds like a whooping crane; child may become cyanotic during episode; mucous plug may be expelled during coughing episode, often followed by vomiting. Apnea often presenting sign in infants under 6 months — persistent cough in older children and adults is often most frequent clinical manifestation.

h. **Diagnostic Procedures** — Positive aspiration culture of nasopharyngeal mucous.

i. **Medical Interventions**

- **Medications** — Erythromycin, clarithromycin; albuterol and corticosteroids may help relieve cough
- **Treatments** — Hospitalization for infants and severely ill, monitor oxygen level, isolation, palliative treatment
- **Surgery** — None necessary

j. **Nursing Interventions** — Isolate child, bedrest with quiet environment, humidified air, increase fluid intake, monitor airway, provide humidified oxygen, administer medication, be alert for signs of respiratory distress.

k. **Potential Complications** — Pneumonia, malnutrition, seizures, rectal prolapse, may cause death if severe obstruction occurs.

3. SCARLET FEVER

a. **Agent** — Group A streptococcal (GAS) infection.

b. **At Risk** — All ages, children 6-12 highest incidence.

c. **Incubation** — Strep pharyngitis: 2-5 days; impetigo: 7-10 days.

d. **Communicable Period** — Variable. Strep pharyngitis: greater during acute respiratory symptoms until after 24 hours of oral antibiotics; impetigo: contagious while lesions draining until treated and dry.

e. **Seasonal Incidence** — Winter and early spring more common.

f. **Transmission** — Contact with infected person or respiratory secretions, may also contract through infected articles, food, skin.

g. **Signs and Symptoms** — Strep pharyngitis: initially high fever, fine red maculopapular rash (blanches with pressure) often concentrated in areas near folds (groin, axilla, neck), fine yellow-red "sandpaper" rash on chest, enlarged red tonsils covered with exudate, white coated tongue progressing to red strawberry tongue, rash desquamates in 1 week; also, cervical adenopathy, headache, nausea and abdominal pain; impetigo: honey colored crusts generally found around the nose and mouth, spread to other areas.

h. **Diagnostic Procedures** — Clinical findings, positive GAS throat or skin culture, positive streptozyme, elevated ASO or Anti-DNase B.

i. **Medical Interventions**
   - **Medication** — GAS pharyngitis: penicillin V, amoxicillin, IM benzathine penicillin, erythromycin, cephalosporins, clindamycin. GAS impetigo: topical anti-bacterial preparations (bacitracin, mupirocin) for few lesions; for multiple lesions systemic antibiotics given. Invasive GAS infection (toxic shock) requires IV antibiotics and immune globulin
   - **Treatment** — Isolation, handwashing, palliative care; hospitalization if severe

j. **Nursing Interventions** — Antibiotic administration, respiratory isolation, bedrest, oral hygiene, increase fluid intake, antipyretics prn, handwashing, teach parents to cleanse and clean impetigo lesions—use separate wash cloth and towel for infected child.

k. **Potential Complications** — Early detection and treatment may reduce these: cervical adenitis, otitis media, sinusitis, pneumonia, rheumatic fever, glomerulonephritis, septicemia, toxic shock.

4. TETANUS ("LOCKJAW")

a. **Agent** — *Clostridium tetani.*

b. **At Risk** — All unimmunized individuals or those with immunizations overdue who experience a wound contaminated by an infective agent; individuals with puncture wounds, extensive burns, or tissue injury are at risk; individuals in rural areas are at higher risk.

   c. **Incubation** — 3-14 days.

   d. **Communicable Period** — Not transmissible from person to person.

   e. **Seasonal Incidence** — Year-round.

   f. **Transmission** — Inanimate objects, soil; dust-carrying organisms which infect susceptible wound.

   g. **Signs and Symptoms** — Initially, muscle stiffness in neck and jaw, progresses to difficulty with swallowing and opening mouth; 24 hours after onset of symptoms, muscles progressively become sensitive to any stimuli; death may result due to respiratory spasm.

   h. **Diagnostic Procedures** — Clinical findings and infrequently a positive wound culture.

   i. **Medical Interventions**
- **Medication** — Tetanus immune globulin (TIG), if TIG not available give intravenous immune globulin (IVIG); administer penicillin G, metronidazole, erythromycin, or tetracycline; control tetany with diazepam, magnesium sulfate, dantrolene, baclofen, vecuronium, pancuronium
- **Treatments** — May require endotracheal intubation or tracheostomy, cardiorespiratory monitoring, suctioning
- **Surgery** — Possible foreign body removal, wound debridement, tracheostomy

   j. **Nursing Interventions** — Prevention through updated immunizations; if last immunization was within 5 years, cleanse wound as needed; if last immunization was within 10 years, administer toxoid booster and cleanse wound; if immunization greater than 10 years old, give toxoid and immunoglobulin and cleanse wound. Monitor VS and monitor for muscle spasms, respiratory distress, I&O, and careful mouth, skin, bowel, bladder care.

   k. **Potential Complications** — Pulmonary spasms, laryngospasm, intra-muscular hematomas, fractures, venous thrombosis, pulmonary embolism, cardiac arrhythmia, labile BP, cerebral palsy, decreased mental functioning, death.

Parasitic Infestations

1. **ENTEROBIASIS (PINWORMS)**

   a. **Agent** — *Enterobius vermicularis.*

   b. **At Risk** — All ages, especially those in crowded living conditions.

   c. **Incubation** — 2 to 4 weeks.

   d. **Communicable Period** — Anytime child is infected; child continues to reinfect self; eggs persist in environment and air for 1 week or longer.

e. **Seasonal Incidence** — Year-round, more common in summer.

f. **Transmission** — Fecal-oral route of ova.

g. **Signs and Symptoms** — Pruritis of anal area, especially at night; may experience anorexia, vulvitis and vaginitis, bedwetting, restlessness, irritability.

h. **Diagnostic Procedures** — Detected by placing clear cellophane tape over anal opening at night, removing and microscopically examining for the presence of ova or worms.

i. **Medical Interventions**
   - **Medication** — Pyrantel pamoate, mebendazole (over 2 years of age only), or piperazine citrate
   - **Treatments** — Treat all household members and re-treat in two weeks as needed
   - **Surgery** — None necessary

j. **Nursing Interventions** — Administer medication as ordered, encourage frequent handwashing especially after diaper change or using the toilet, and before eating. Keep diapers in a closed container, encourage showers instead of tub baths. Instruct parents in obtaining tape test for ova, washing linen and clothing in hot soapy water. Vacuum, clean toys and furniture.

k. **Potential Complications** — Secondary infection from scratching.

2. **PEDICULOSIS CAPITUS (HEAD LICE)**

a. **Agent** — *Pediculosis humanus capitus.*

b. **At Risk** — All ages, anytime.

c. **Incubation** — 7 to 10 days.

d. **Communicable Period** — Anytime eggs or live lice present on individual.

e. **Seasonal Incidence** — Year-round.

f. **Transmission** — Fingernails; shared inanimate objects containing nits and lice such as hairbrushes, combs, hats, bedding, clothing, toys.

g. **Signs and Symptoms** — Itching of scalp; white balls or salt-like nit cases on hair shaft, especially around nape of neck and behind ears; visible lice, cervical and occipital adenopathy, scratch marks and inflammatory papules.

h. **Diagnostic Procedures** — Clinical findings.

i. **Medical Interventions**
   - **Medication** — Permethrin 1%, pyrethrin shampoo, or 1% lindane shampoo
   - **Treatments** — Treat all family members, repeat medication in one week if needed
   - **Surgery** — None necessary

    j. Nursing Interventions — Isolate from school or day care; check hair, eyebrows and eyelashes carefully; use peduculicidal shampoo or cream rinse as instructed, comb out nits, repeat application in one week; encourage handwashing; launder linens and clothing in hot soapy water or dry clean; discard or clean all hair items in a pediculicide.

    k. Potential Complications — Secondary infection due to scratching.

3. SCABIES

    a. Agent — *Sarcoptes scabei hominis.*

    b. At Risk — All ages.

    c. Incubation — 30-60 days from infestation to onset of symptoms.

    d. Communicable Period — Entire time individual is infested.

    e. Seasonal Incidence — Year-round.

    f. Transmission — Prolonged contact (greater than 45 minutes) with infected individual.

    g. Signs and Symptoms — Under 2 years of age: largest amount of eruptions on palms, soles, face, scalp, burrows often absent and bullae and pustules common; older children and adolescents have lesions following axillary lines, inner aspect of upper arm, interdigital webs, ankles, wrists; lesions may have thread-like burrows; lesions at all ages are intensely pruritic, lymphadenopathy at regional site of lesions.

    h. Diagnostic Procedures — Clinical findings, microscopic identification of mites collected from a skin scraping.

    i. Medical Interventions

      – **Medication** — Lindane cream 1%, Permethrin 5% (use in infants); antibiotics if secondary infection

      – **Treatments** — May need to treat all persons in contact due to long time between infestation and development of symptoms

      – **Surgery** — None necessary

    j. Nursing Interventions — Apply topical lotion as directed from neck down and under fingernails; launder all recently worn clothing, bed linens in hot soapy water or dry clean; wear gloves; encourage hand washing; be alert for signs of medication toxicity: nausea, vomiting, weakness, tremors, irritability, seizures, respiratory distress.

    k. Potential Complications — Infection secondary to scratching, cellulitis, lymphangitis, possible glomerulonephritis as a result of secondary streptococcal infection of lesions, neurotoxicity of medications.

Viral Infections

1. ### ERYTHEMA INFECTIOSUM (FIFTH'S DISEASE)
   a. **Agent** — *Human parvovirus.*
   b. **At Risk** — Usually children 6-10 years old; harmful to fetuses.
   c. **Incubation** — 4-21 days.
   d. **Communicable Period** — Unknown; most likely before onset of symptoms and for the first 1-2 days of the rash.
   e. **Seasonal Incidence** — Most common in winter and spring and occurs in cyclical patterns that peak about every 6 years.
   f. **Transmission** — Direct contact with respiratory droplets, blood.
   g. **Signs and Symptoms** — Staged rash: initially begins with mild muscle/joint aches, low-grade fever, sore throat, headache followed by erythema on face ("slapped cheek"); appearance lasting 1-4 days; progresses to maculopapular rash on all extremities starting proximally, lasting 7 or more days; in stage III the rash subsides and becomes lace-like; rash can reappear with stress, sunlight exposure, exercise, and temperature changes; rash lasts total of 2-3 weeks, spares the palms and soles, and is mildly pruritic in older children.
   h. **Diagnostic Procedures** — Clinical findings, serum B19 specific IgM antibody can be done if needed.
   i. **Medical Interventions**
      – **Medications** — Antipyretics, antipruritic if needed
      – **Treatments** — Palliative care
      – **Surgery** — None necessary
   j. **Nursing Interventions** — Supportive care of parent and child, infection usually self-limiting; administer antipyretics and antipruritics as needed; isolate immunocompromised patients; advise pregnant women of the potential risk.
   k. **Potential Complications** — Atypical but may experience arthritic symptoms; children with blood dyscrasias may develop aplastic anemia, chronic infections of erythema infectiosum; aseptic meningitis, thrombocytopenia purpura; potential risk of fetal hydrops and death if mother infected during pregnancy.

2. ### EXANTHEM SUBITUM (ROSEOLA INFANTUM)
   a. **Agent** — *Human herpesvirus type 6 (HHV — 6)* in 80-90% of cases.
   b. **At Risk** — Children 6 months to 4 years (90% by 2 years of age).
   c. **Incubation** — 5 to 15 days.
   d. **Communicable Period** — Uncertain.
   e. **Seasonal Incidence** — Year-round, higher incidence in spring and summer.

f. **Transmission** — Unknown; most likely respiratory droplet.

g. **Signs and Symptoms** — High fever for 3-4 days (39°C to 41°C), followed by appearance of maculopapular rose-pink rash first on trunk then neck, face, and extremities (lasts for 1-3 days); may have URI symptoms, cervical/occipital adenopathy.

h. **Diagnostic Procedures** — None required, may have a CBC to help with diagnosis; WBC may be 16,000-20,000 mm^3 for first 24 hours of fever; leukopenia develops within 3-5 days.

i. **Medical Interventions**
   - **Medications** — Antipyretics, sedatives for children prone to seizures
   - **Treatments** — Palliative
   - **Surgery** — None necessary

j. **Nursing Interventions** — Assist parents with methods to control fever, discuss seizure precautions and measures; provide parents with information describing this benign infection; administer antipyretics as needed; be alert to signs of seizure activity.

k. **Potential Complications** — Febrile seizures (can be prevented), encephalitis (rare), multi-organ failure in immunosuppressed child.

3. **MEASLES (RUBEOLA)**

   a. **Agent** — *Morbillivirus.*

   b. **At Risk** — Any unimmunized person, particularly preschool, adolescents, young adults.

   c. **Incubation** — 8 to 20 days.

   d. **Communicable Period** — 2 to 4 days prior to onset of symptoms until 5 days after onset of rash.

   e. **Seasonal Incidence** — Winter and spring.

   f. **Transmission** — Respiratory droplets, blood, urine of infected person.

   g. **Signs and Symptoms** — Prodromal stage: begins as an upper respiratory infection with fever, malaise, cough, sore throat, Koplik spots, and conjunctivitis; the temperature rises as the maculopapular rash appears 4-5 days after onset of respiratory symptoms; begins on face (around hairline and neck) and spreads to trunk and extremities. The rash is often confluent and hemorrhagic and involves the palms and soles; rash typically subsides in 7-10 days; as the rash fades it becomes brownish and begins to desquamate; usually severe photophobia accompanies the conjunctivitis and small children may have gastrointestinal symptoms.

   h. **Diagnostic Procedures** — Clinical findings; positive culture of nasopharyngeal secretions, blood, or urine; positive measles specific IgM antibodies in serum.

   i. **Medical Interventions**
      - **Medication** — Gamma globulin in high risk children; antipyretics, antibiotics if secondary infection

       – **Treatments** — Palliative

       – **Surgery** — None necessary

  j. Nursing Interventions — Prevention through adequate immunization, treat symptoms as needed, fever management, isolation until noncontagious, eye care and protection from light, maintain hydration, cool humidity for cough, be alert to signs of complications.

  k. Potential Complications — Otitis media, pneumonia, encephalitis bronchiolitis, myocarditis.

4. MONONUCLEOSIS

  a. Agent — *Epstein-Barr virus (EBV).*

  b. At Risk — Adolescents and young adults, occurs at any age.

  c. Incubation — 4 to 6 weeks.

  d. Communicable Period — Unknown.

  e. Seasonal Incidence — Year-round.

  f. Transmission — Oropharyngeal secretions or intimate contact, blood transfusion, organ transplant.

  g. Signs and Symptoms — Headache, anorexia, malaise, extreme fatigue, moderate fever, sore throat, exudate on tonsils, generalized lymphadenopathy, hepatosplenomegaly, maculopapular rash.

  h. Diagnostic Procedures — Clinical findings, positive serologic tests EBV specific, positive monospot agglutination test, positive heterophile antibody test.

  i. Medical Interventions

       – **Medication** — Antipyretics, corticosteroids if severe respiratory distress, antibiotics if secondary infection (avoid penicillin and amoxicillin as they precipitate a rash)

       – **Treatments** — Palliative, avoid contact sports for 6-8 weeks due to the spleen and liver enlargement

       – **Surgery** — None necessary

  j. Nursing Interventions — Comfort measures, bedrest, increase fluids, administer corticosteroids, antipyretics, and antibiotics as prescribed, encourage good nutrition; teach individual and parents that rest is essential, may have recurrence of symptoms; fatigue can persist for months.

  k. Potential Complications — Secondary infections, myocarditis, hemolytic anemia, ruptured spleen, liver damage, airway obstruction due to edema of airway.

5. MUMPS (PAROTITIS)

  a. Agent — *Paramyxovirus.*

  b. At Risk — Any unvaccinated person, all people susceptible, highest incidence in 1-14 year olds.

   c. **Incubation** — 14-24 days.

   d. **Communicable Period** — Uncertain but thought to be 1 to 2 days before and 3 to 4 days after swelling phase.

   e. **Seasonal Incidence** — Year-round, more common winter and spring.

   f. **Transmission** — Through saliva of infected person.

   g. **Signs and Symptoms** — Initially headache, low-grade fever, malaise, anorexia, localized pain around ear and jawline, usually swelling of only one parotid gland, may be quite painful, usually resolves in 3-7 days; parotitis can be caused by other organisms, so can recur.

   h. **Diagnostic Procedures** — Clinical findings, positive serologic antibodies, positive viral culture of saliva, urine, blood or cerebral spinal fluid.

   i. **Medical Interventions**
      – **Medications** — Antipyretics
      – **Treatments** — Palliative
      – **Surgery** — None necessary

   j. **Nursing Interventions** — Prevent through vaccination; bedrest; isolation; analgesics, antipyretics as needed; soft or blended foods, avoid sour foods; increased fluid intake; support genitalia.

   k. **Potential Complications** — Epidydimo-orchiditis, deafness, encephalitis, myocarditis, hepatitis, neuritis, arthritis, sterility.

6. **POLIOMYELITIS**

   a. **Agent** — *Enteroviruses Type 1, 2, 3.*

   b. **At Risk** — Any unvaccinated person, more common in infants and very young children.

   c. **Incubation** — 7-14 days with a range of 3-35 days.

   d. **Communicable Period** — 3-5 days after exposure until 6-8 weeks after symptoms appear.

   e. **Seasonal Incidence** — Summer and early fall.

   f. **Transmission** — Contact with stool, salivary secretions, or blood of infected person.

   g. **Signs and Symptoms** — May take one of four forms:
      – Asymptomatic
      – Abortive poliomyelitis: fever, sore throat, headache, abdominal pain, nausea and vomiting, malaise
      – Nonparalytic poliomyelitis: more severe symptoms as above accompanied by stiffness in back, neck, and legs, bulging fontanel in infants, constipation, bladder paralysis
      – Paralytic poliomyelitis: symptoms as listed in previous forms, progresses to apparent signs of CNS involvement

    h. **Diagnostic Procedures** — Culture of feces, pharynx, urine or CSF.

    i. **Medical Interventions**

       – **Medications** — Analgesics, sedatives, bladder stimulants (bethanechol)

       – **Treatments** — Hot packs to muscles, physical therapy, splinting, positioning to maintain position of function, hydration with IV fluids, respirator if impaired respiratory function

       – **Surgery** — Tracheostomy may be needed

    j. **Nursing Interventions** — Treat symptoms as they occur, utilize isolation and enteric precautions, bedrest, PT exercises as indicated, observe for signs of paralysis and which systems are affected, monitor BP, I&O, encourage fluids and manage constipation with diet and supplements as needed; monitor for signs of respiratory impairment: restlessness, irritability, poor feeding, fatigue, anxiety.

    k. **Potential Complications** — Paralysis (temporary or long-term), respiratory difficulties or arrest, hypertension, death.

7. **RUBELLA (GERMAN MEASLES)**

    a. **Agent** — *Rubivirus.*

    b. **At Risk** — Any unimmunized person, unborn fetus at high risk for birth defects; peak age of disease in teenagers and young adults.

    c. **Incubation** — 14-21 days.

    d. **Communicable Period** — From 7 days before symptoms to 5 days after rash appears.

    e. **Seasonal Incidence** — Spring more common.

    f. **Transmission** — Airborne droplets from respiratory secretions, contaminated articles, feces, urine of infected person.

    g. **Signs and Symptoms** — May be asymptomatic, low-grade fever, malaise, anorexia, occipital, posterior auricular, and cervical adenopathy; discrete maculopapules and flushing beginning on the face and progressing to the trunk with coalescence; pinpoint papules may appear on the trunk, mild pruritis, rash disappears in the same sequence as appearance by day 3-4.

    h. **Diagnostic Procedures** — Viral culture of nasopharynx, elevated rubella antibody titers (obtain acute and convalescent).

    i. **Medical Interventions**

       – **Medication** — None

       – **Treatments** — Palliative

       – **Surgery** — None necessary

    j. **Nursing Interventions** — Keep pregnant women in first trimester away from infected child, treat symptoms as needed; do not give live vaccine to pregnant women.

    k. **Potential Complications** — Rare, but can have arthritis, encephalitis, purpura, congenital rubella syndrome (fetus).

8. VARICELLA ZOSTER (CHICKENPOX)

a. **Agent** — *Varicella zoster virus (VZV).*

b. **At Risk** — Typically seen in children 2-8 years old, can be any age. High risk children: CF, diabetes, salycilate therapy, immunocompromised.

c. **Incubation** — 7-21 days.

d. **Communicable Period** — 1- 2 days prior to skin eruptions and until all lesions have scabbed over and there are no new lesions.

e. **Seasonal Incidence** — Higher in winter and spring.

f. **Transmission** — Direct contact with contagious person, respiratory droplets, contaminated inanimate objects.

g. **Signs and Symptoms** — Low-grade fever, rash which progresses from macules to papules to vesicles and then lesions scab; lesions spread from trunk to extremities and face (papule, vesicle, crust lesions present at same time); intense itching.

h. **Diagnostic Procedures** — Clinical findings, immunofluorescent staining of vesicular scrapings show VZV, acute and convalescent antibody serologic tests.

i. **Medical Interventions**

   – **Medications** — For children who are immunosuppressed or high risk (CF, diabetes, children on salycilate therapy) give acyclovir within 24 hours after exposure to infected individual; varicella zoster immune globulin (VZIG) given to high risk children, pregnant women, immunosuppressed individuals; use acetamenophen for analgesic, antipyretic; also antipruritic agents topically (calamine) and orally (diphenhydramine hydrocloride); antibiotics for secondary infection; avoid aspirin due to the risk of Reye's Syndrome

   – **Treatments** — Palliative

   – **Surgery** — None necessary

j. **Nursing Interventions** — Comfort care to decrease pruritis and secondary infections due to itching; isolate child until scabs have covered all lesions, keep fingernails short and clean, bathe in baking soda or oatmeal. Be alert to signs of infections, complications.

k. **Potential Complications** — Scarring, secondary bacterial infections, encephalitis, pneumonia, herpes zoster.

10

INTEGUMENTARY DISORDERS

I. General Concepts

- The skin functions to regulate heat, provide a means for sensation, protect the body from invading organisms, and prevent desiccation of the underlying structures

- The skin is composed of the epidermis, dermis, subcutaneous tissues and accessory structures (hair, fingernails, sweat glands, sebaceous glands)

- The skin changes as the infant grows and develops; the epidermis is not adherent to the dermis initially in infancy and this allows for easier blistering; the pH changes from acidic to alkaline with age; sebaceous glands are active initially at birth then decrease activity until adolescence

- Skin disorders may be acute or chronic and require treatment to prevent secondary infections

II. Specific Integumentary Disorder

Acquired Disorders

1. ACNE VULGARIS

   a. **Description** — The presence of comedones (blackheads and whiteheads) and pustules that are typically located on the face, chest, and back. It is due to plugging of the sebaceous glands. It is most commonly seen in adolescence as the sebaceous glands become more active.

b. **Signs and Symptoms** — Lesions: blackheads (open comedones), whiteheads (closed comedones), and pustules with inflammation.

c. **Diagnostic Procedures** — Diagnosed by characteristic physical findings.

d. **Medical Interventions**
   - **Medications** — Application of topical ketolytic (RetinA, Benzoyl peroxide), systemic or topical antibiotic therapy (Tetracycline, Clindamycin), and/or oral retinoids (Accutane)
   - **Treatment** — Focuses on keeping area clean, comedone removal (in some cases), ultraviolet light therapy and estrogen therapy (in some cases)
   - **Surgery** — Unnecessary

e. **Nursing Interventions**
   - **Assessment and Actions**
     * Assess for any areas of inflammation or secondary infection
     * Discourage vigorous scrubbing or "picking" at the lesions
     * Assess for signs indicating potential complications
   - **Teaching**
     * Explain cause and treatment regimen with adolescent and parents; include a written, detailed description of the home treatment schedule
     * Instruct teen to keep areas clean and to maintain good hygiene in susceptible areas; wash face and/or other affected areas with warm, soapy water no more than three times per day for one minute; rinse well, use a clean washcloth each time
     * Instruct teen on avoiding sun exposure after ultraviolet light therapy or oral retinoids
     * Teach parents and teen about medications prescribed (drug, dose, route, and side effects)
     * Advise that condition usually worsens before it improves
   - **Emotional Care**
     * Discuss how teen sees self and promote teen's self-esteem
     * Inform of typical improvement of acne with age
     * Provide support to family and teen

f. **Complications** — Scarring, secondary infections.

2. **ATOPIC DERMATITIS (ECZEMA)**
   a. **Description** - Superficial dermatitis that occurs in all age groups but occurs most frequently in infants and young children. It typically begins as pruritic, erythematous, papulovesicular lesions and progresses to crusty, thickened areas. The sites that are frequently affected include cheeks and joints of arms and legs. The etiology is

unknown but is thought to be an allergic response. There may be a history of asthma or hayfever in the family.

b. **Signs and Symptoms** — Erythematous, pruritic, papulovesicular lesions followed by scabbing and crust formation in area, then thickening of the skin.

c. **Diagnostic Procedures** — Diagnosed by characteristic physical findings and associated family history.

d. **Medical Interventions**
   - **Medications** — Administration of antihistamines, antibiotics (systemic), or topical corticosteroids (Synlar)
   - **Treatments** — Focuses on identification of allergen, modification or removal of source of irritation, prevention of secondary infection, application of moist dressings, avoidance of harsh soaps, application of lanolin-based or oil-in-water-based emulsions immediately after bathing to seal in moisture
   - **Surgery** — Unnecessary

e. **Nursing Interventions**
   - **Assessment and Actions**
     * Record assessment findings to monitor progress
     * Assist with determining potential causes and eliminate from environment if possible
     * Provide method for reducing discomfort
     * Assess for signs indicating potential complications
   - **Teaching**
     * Explain diagnosis and discuss treatment regimen with family and child
     * Instruct family on keeping area clean, avoiding hot water to area, taking short baths, applying nonlipid lotions to area, and preventing scratching by cutting fingernails and using over-the-counter medications, such as diphenhydramine, to diminish pruritus
     * Teach parents about medication prescribed (drug, dose, route, time, and side effects)
   - **Emotional Care**
     * Provide support to family and child since itching and discomfort associated with eczema can cause the infant or child to be very irritable

f. **Potential Complications** — Secondary infections, scarring.

3. **BURNS**

   a. **Description** — Injury to any layer of the skin caused by thermal, chemical, electrical sources, or overexposure to ultraviolet rays.

b. **Signs and Symptoms** — Depend upon severity:
  - **Superficial-partial thickness burn** (first degree: epidermis) exhibits redness and tenderness of area similar to a sunburn; the wound blanches with pressure
  - **Partial-thickness burn** (second degree: epidermis and dermis) causes severe pain; area is reddened, is usually moist, blanches with pressure and may be blistered
  - **Full-thickness burn** (third degree: all regenerative elements in the dermis and epidermis are destroyed) is dry, may appear white or leathery, usually lacks sensation and no blanching occurs; in black children with third degree injury, the skin may look similar to skin of unburned Caucasian children due to destruction of melanin
  - **Full-thickness burn** (fourth degree) extends below the dermis to underlying structures such as bone and muscle

c. **Diagnostic Procedures** — Diagnosed by obtaining history of injury and physical findings.

d. **Medical Interventions**
  - **Medications** — Application of topical antibiotics and IV antibiotics
  - **Treatments** — Treatment depends upon severity, extent and area; superficial-partial thickness burns are typically treated at home by keeping area cleansed, providing fluids and promoting rest; partial-thickness and full-thickness burns are treated by cleaning area several times each day, applying topical antibiotic ointments as ordered, monitoring vital signs, fluid status, urine output, respiratory status, circulation to area, providing pain control, assessing bowel sounds, promoting nutrition, grafting area and providing physical therapy once healed
  - **Surgery** — Escharotomy, skin grafting, or amputation may be necessary

e. **Nursing Interventions**
  - **Assessment and Actions**
    * Obtain vital signs, weight, height and history of injury
    * Monitor respirations and maintain patent airway especially if injured in closed space or soot present around mouth or nose
    * Provide method for reducing discomfort
    * If hospitalization required, monitor: vital signs, airway patency, fluid and electrolyte status, I&O, nutritional intake, circulation to distal area of burn, respiratory status, and bowel sounds; utilize sterile technique for all procedures, document change in wound(s) with each dressing change, position to promote function of injured area (especially joints); place NG tube
    * Administer antibiotics and other medications as ordered
    * Encourage child to perform own ADLs as able
    * Facilitate referral (PT, OT, social workers)
    * Assess for signs indicating potential complications

- **Teaching**
  * Explain injury to parents and child and discuss treatment regimen
  * If care is to be given at home, teach caregiver how to care for area and about the signs and symptoms which require further medical assistance
  * If surgery is required, explain procedures to parents and child and plan of care before, during, and after procedure
  * Ensure proper discharge planning allowing appropriate time for instruction and return demonstration of wound care and physical therapy
  * Teach parents about medications prescribed (drug, dose, route, time, and side effects)
- **Emotional Care**
  * Encourage parents to be involved with child's care as allowed
  * Promote growth and development while hospitalized
  * Promote child's self-esteem and discuss change in body and body image
  * Discuss anxiety about treatment and alteration in appearance
  * Provide support to family and child during and after hospitalization

f. **Potential Complications** — Depend on severity, extent, depth and area of injury but may include infection, contractions, scarring, paralytic ileus, renal failure, shock, acidosis, respiratory failure, loss of limb(s), death.

4. **CELLULITIS**

   a. **Description** — An infection of the skin located in the dermis or subcutaneous tissue. It is usually caused by *Staphylococcus aureus*, *Group A beta-hemolytic streptococci*, or *Hemophilus influenza*.

   b. **Signs and Symptoms** — Redness, swelling, warmth, induration, and tenderness in area, fever, malaise, lymphangitis; often located in the periorbital area, cheeks, or arms.

   c. **Diagnostic Procedures** — Diagnosed by physical findings and history; blood cultures or aspiration may be performed to identify organism; x-ray may be utilized to rule out osteomyelitis.

   d. **Medical Interventions**
      - **Medications** — Administer organism-specific antibiotic; aggressive antibiotic therapy is warranted in periorbital cellulitis because of potential for brain abscess
      - **Treatments** — Apply warm compresses, immobilize area
      - **Surgery** — Unnecessary unless area becomes necrotic

   e. **Nursing Interventions**
      - **Assessment and Actions**
        * Be alert to signs and symptoms indicating disorder

* Monitor and record changes in appearance of skin
* If nonresponsive to oral antibiotics, prepare child and family for hospitalization for IV administration
* Provide method for reducing discomfort
* Assess for signs indicating potential complications

- **Teaching**
  * Explain diagnosis to parents and child and discuss treatment regimen
  * Teach parents to keep area immobilized and apply warm soaks to area
  * Teach parents about medications prescribed (drug, dose, route, time, and side effects)
- **Emotional Care**
  * Provide support to family and child

f. **Potential Complications** — Systemic infection.

5. **DIAPER DERMATITIS (DIAPER RASH)**

a. **Description** — The presence of erythematous lesions and maceration in the diaper area that is due to prolonged contact with urine, feces, chemical irritants, bacterial or fungal infections, or reactions to certain foods.

b. **Signs and Symptoms** — Erythematous lesions which cause discomfort in diaper area.

c. **Diagnostic Procedures** — Diagnosed by physical findings; rule out fungal and ammoniacal diaper rash which have papules and vesicles.

d. **Medical Interventions**
- **Medications** — Apply topical ointments (Desitin, A&D ointments), topical glucocorticoid or, if fungal infection is present, application of Nystatin ointment
- **Treatments** — Remove irritant, keeping area clean and dry
- **Surgery** — Unnecessary

e. **Nursing Interventions**
- **Assessment and Actions**
  * Be alert to signs and symptoms
  * Provide method for reducing discomfort
  * Assess for signs indicating potential complications
- **Teaching**
  * Explain diagnosis to parents and discuss treatment regimen which includes:
    - Assisting with identifying irritant
    - Discussing importance of keeping area dry and clean
    - Encouraging prompt changing and cleansing of area after each voiding and stool, using mild soap and water

- Avoiding the use of alcohol-based baby wipes
- Allowing area to air dry in between changing times
- Applying ointment to area after cleansed
- Assessing area with each diaper change for signs of worsening or improvement
- Discouraging the use of plastic pants

  — **Emotional Care**

    * Provide support to family and reassure infant's irritability will diminish as area heals

 f. **Potential Complications** — Discomfort and secondary infections.

6. **DRUG-INDUCED SKIN REACTION**

  a. **Description** — An allergic reaction to a topical or systemic medication.

  b. **Signs and Symptoms** — Erythematous and/or urticarial lesions that may be localized or may be widespread depending on route of medication; wheezing; reaction may cause pruritus, fever, and if severe, respiratory distress and anaphylactic shock.

  c. **Diagnostic Procedures** — Diagnosed by reviewing history and physical findings.

  d. **Medical Interventions**

   — **Medications** — Administer antihistamine and/or corticosteroid; monitor for anaphylactic shock

   — **Treatments** — Remove or discontinue use of irritant

   — **Surgery** — Unnecessary

  e. **Nursing Interventions**

   — **Assessment and Actions**

    * Assess child prior to administration of any medication for known allergies and previous response

    * Observe for signs of reaction and discontinue medication immediately if reaction occurs

    * Monitor child's vital signs, record reaction symptoms and signs and observe for signs of anaphylactic reaction

    * Treat pruritus and rash with antihistamines and steroids as ordered

    * Assess for signs indicating potential complications

   — **Teaching**

    * Discuss reaction with family and importance of telling future medical teams about reaction

    * Encourage child to wear a Medic Alert bracelet or tag

    * Teach parents about reaction, how to prevent and treat

    * Teach parents about medications prescribed (drug, dose, route, time, and side effects) and when to use

- **Emotional Care**
  * Provide support to family and child during treatment regimen
f. **Potential Complications** — Anaphylactic reaction.

7. **IMPETIGO**

a. **Description** — A superficial infection of the skin due to invasion by staphylococcal or streptococcal organisms. It typically begins as a scratch that becomes infected. It may be transmitted to others by direct contact with lesion or drainage from lesion. It is usually seen in the infant and toddler age groups and is the most contagious and most common skin infection seen in children.

b. **Signs and Symptoms** — Begins as discrete erythematous area around dirty scratch; lesion then forms small vesicles that break and release a honey-colored fluid which forms a crust or scab; typically found around mouth, cheeks, face, (especially across the nose) or hands, but may spread over any part of the body.

c. **Diagnostic Procedures** — Diagnosed by characteristic findings and positive culture of vesicular fluid.

d. **Medical Interventions**
   - **Medications** — May apply antibacterial ointment, and possibly administer systemic antibiotic therapy (penicillin or dicloxacillin) if severe
   - **Treatments** — Cleanse area, remove crusts with compresses soaked with Burow's solution (astringent solution of aluminum acetate) or warm water and soap; cleaning the lesions is important to prevent secondary infection
   - **Surgery** — Unnecessary

e. **Nursing Interventions**
   - **Assessment and Actions**
     * Be alert to signs and symptoms
     * Document appearance, size, and location of lesions
     * Provide method for reducing discomfort
     * Assess for signs indicating potential complication
   - **Teaching**
     * Explain diagnosis to parents
     * Instruct parents on treatment regimen:
       - Cleanse area with Burow's solution as ordered
       - Soak areas that have crusting and scabbing before removal
       - Apply antibacterial ointment as ordered
       - Prevent scratching of area by child
       - If lesions do not improve, discuss need for systemic antibiotic therapy
       - Emphasize communicability of infection and importance of maintaining good hygiene for child and thorough handwashing for caregiver

- Teach parents about medications prescribed (drug, dose, route, time, and side effects)

   – **Emotional Care**

     * Provide support to family and child and reassure that disorder can usually be treated at home without complications

  f. **Potential Complications** — Scarring, acute glomerulonephritis if left untreated.

8. **SEBORRHEIC DERMATITIS**

  a. **Description** — Erythematous areas of the skin that are due to an excess discharge from the sebaceous glands. It is typically found on the scalp and eyebrows. It is known as cradle cap in infancy and may also be present in adolescence.

  b. **Signs and Symptoms** — Patchy lesions on the scalp or eyebrows which are covered by yellowish, oily scales; area may become macerated and ooze if left untreated.

  c. **Diagnostic Procedures** — Diagnosed by characteristic physical findings.

  d. **Medical Interventions**

    – **Medications** — Apply mineral oil to infant's scalp, utilize antiseborrheic shampoo, apply topical steroid and/or antibiotics (in some instances)

    – **Treatments** — Improve hygiene to area

    – **Surgery** — Not applicable

  e. **Nursing Interventions**

    – **Assessment and Actions**

     * Be alert to signs and symptoms indicating disorder

     * Document appearance, size, and locations of lesions

     * Determine whether treatment is effective (severe cases may require antiseptic shampoo, topical steroids, and antibiotic therapy)

     * Assess for signs indicating potential complications

    – **Teaching**

     * Discuss treatment regimen with parents and child:

      - Emphasize importance of washing scalp thoroughly with shampoo including the fontanelle in infants (which the parent may be afraid of doing) and rinsing area thoroughly

      - Apply and massage mineral oil on affected area 15 minutes prior to washing infant's scalp to loosen up scales

      - Comb out scales after shampooing

    – **Emotional Care**

     * Provide support to parents and child and emphasize that cases are simply treated at home and usually resolve

  f. **Potential Complications** — Secondary infection to area if left untreated.

9. **TINEA CAPITIS OR CORPORIS (RINGWORM OF SCALP OR BODY)**

   a. **Description** — The presence of a fungal infection on the scalp (tinea capitis) or body (tinea corporis).

   b. **Signs and Symptoms** — Scaly, round or oval erythematous patches on the scalp (capitis) or on the body (corporis); pruritus, and alopecia with broken hair shafts (tinea capitis).

   c. **Diagnostic Procedures** — Diagnosed by utilizing Wood's lamp (sites appear green) and KOH smears (reveals spores).

   d. **Medical Interventions**

      – **Medications** — Topical antifungals (econazole, miconazole or clotrimazole) applied for two weeks, twice a day; an oral fungicide (griseofulvin) is usually given if the condition responds poorly to topical fungicides

      – **Treatments** — Frequent shampooing of hair; selenium sulfide shampoo is used twice a week (tinea capitis); keep skin dry and clean (tinea corporis)

      – **Surgery** — Unnecessary

   e. **Nursing Interventions**

      – **Assessment and Actions**

         * Be alert to signs and symptoms

         * Document appearance, size, and location of lesion

         * Recheck scalp and body after 2 weeks to ensure fungus is gone

         * Assess for signs indicating potential complications

      – **Teaching**

         * Discuss treatment regimen with family and importance of taking/applying medication regularly

         * Instruct about importance of thorough washing of hair, scalp (tinea capitis) and body every day

         * Teach parents about medication prescribed (drug, dose, route, time, and side effects)

         * Teach parents that heat and moisture enhance the fungal infection; infected areas must be kept dry

      – **Emotional Care**

         * Discuss alopecia and that hair will grow back in areas once infection treated (tinea capitis)

         * Provide support to family and child

   f. **Potential Complications** — Permanent scarring or baldness if left untreated or treated late (tinea capitis).

11

CENTRAL NERVOUS SYSTEM DISORDERS

I.   General Concepts

- The nervous system is comprised of the central nervous system, autonomic nervous system, and peripheral nervous system

- The nervous system continues to grow and develop after birth and through adolescence

- The central nervous system (CNS) functions to control and regulate the body. It provides a communication network within the body. It receives information from internal and external stimuli and determines the appropriate response to maintain homeostasis

II. Specific Central Nervous System Disorders

Congenital Disorders

1. CEREBRAL PALSY

a. **Description** — A chronic impairment of motor control and muscle tone resulting from a non-progressive abnormality in the pyramidal motor system. It is often associated with perinatal brain ischemia, prematurity, low birth weight, and birth trauma. There are three major types:
   1) Spastic (comprises majority)
   2) Athetoid
   3) Ataxic

b. **Signs and Symptoms** — Depend upon type; general findings include delays and abnormalities in development especially motor control and performance; increased or decreased muscle tone; persistent primitive reflexes; unusual posture; may also exhibit seizure activity, ADD, hyperactivity, mental retardation, and deficits in vision or hearing.

c. **Diagnostic Procedures** — Usually difficult to diagnose until child is 2-4 months or older when neurological exam reveals abnormalities, including impairment of voluntary muscle movement and posturing.

d. **Medical Interventions**
   – **Medications** — May administer anticonvulsant and muscle relaxants (diazepam, dantrolene, baclofen) but often benefits do not outweigh side effects; botulinum toxin, phenol injected as motor point blocks to relieve spasticity
   – **Treatments** — Utilize physical therapy, braces, casts, corrective appliances, glasses, hearing aids, technical aids (computer voice synthesizer)
   – **Surgery** — May require surgical correction of spasticity and contractions (including dorsal rhizotomy), tenotomy of Achilles tendon

e. **Nursing Interventions**
   – **Assessment and Actions**
     * Be alert for signs and symptoms
     * Monitor child for persistent primitive reflexes; delay in gross motor milestones such as head control, sitting, crawling, feeding difficulties; and failure to develop postural reflexes such as equilibrium, stiffness or floppy muscle tone
     * Facilitate referrals to appropriate professional resources (OT, PT) and organizations such as Easter Seals for physical, speech, and occupational therapy, assistance in obtaining special equipment (wheelchairs, car seats)
     * Assess for signs indicating potential complication: aspiration, failure to thrive, recurrent respiratory infections
   – **Teaching**
     * Determine parents' and child's level of understanding of disorder.

* Teach parents and child about disorder, diagnosis, long-term treatments and implications

* Assist parents with learning how to care for child and how to enhance growth and development and ADLs

* Assist parents with determining mode of mobilizing child (wheelchair, braces, walkers), communicating with child, and providing safety for child, including seizure precautions (include provision of safe environment with protection from falls, etc. and may include such interventions as wearing a helmet) and actions to take if seizure occurs

* Teach parents about medication prescribed (drug, dose, route, time, and side effects)

* Instruct parents on ROM and prevention of skin breakdown

  – **Emotional Care**

* Allow for grief response of parents

* Monitor how family is coping with illness

* Provide support to family and child

* Provide support group information to family

f. **Potential Complications** — Delayed growth and development, skin breakdown, contractures, seizures, difficulty with vision, hearing or communicating; may also have various degrees of mental retardation, aspiration pneumonias, failure to thrive.

2. HYDROCEPHALUS

a. **Description** — A problem with over-production, under-absorption or obstruction of flow of CSF in the brain's ventricular circulation. Hydrocephalus may be categorized as communicating or noncommunicating and may be congenital (most common) or acquired.

b. **Signs and Symptoms** — Depend upon age; infants: prior to closure of suture lines may exhibit an enlarged head circumference (macrocephaly), bulging fontanels, Macewen's cracked pot sign, setting sun eyes, lethargy, poor feeding, high pitched cry; children may exhibit headaches, vomiting, irritability, seizures, confusion, and a change in level of consciousness, incoordination, papilledema.

c. **Diagnostic Procedures** — Diagnosed by physical findings; CT scan reveals enlarged ventricles and site of CSF blockage; x-ray reveals enlarged cranium; MRI may reveal Arnold Chiari malformation (downward displacement of lower brain stem, cerebellum, and fourth ventricle into foramen magnum).

d. **Medical Interventions**

  – **Medications** — Administer Isosorbide preoperatively; postoperatively administer acetazolamide, furosemide, antibiotics, anticonvulsant

  – **Treatments** — Monitor for signs of increased intracranial pressure before and after surgery, ventricular taps in infant (until infant is large enough for shunt placement)

- **Surgery** — Surgical placement of Ventriculoperitoneal (V-P) or ventricular-atrial (V-A) shunts and removal of obstruction, when possible

e. **Nursing Interventions**

- **Assessment and Actions**

  * Be alert to signs and symptoms that indicate increased intracranial pressure/hydrocephalus

  * Monitor infant's head circumference and observe for signs of increasing intracranial pressure (see following section on Increased Intracranial Pressure)

  * Preoperatively position infant to prevent skin breakdown and support infant's head when turning from side to side

  * Postoperatively monitor signs, respiratory and neuro status, maintain adequate hydration and nutrition, assess for signs of IICP and signs of infection, measure I&O carefully

  * Assess for signs indicating potential complications: elevated V/S, poor feeding, vomiting, seizures, change in neuro status

- **Teaching**

  * Explain procedures and treatment regimen to parents and child

  * Teach family and child about shunt and how to assess its functioning

  * Inform parents and child of signs of shunt malfunction or increased intracranial pressure and when to call physician

  * Teach parents to "pump" shunt to assess functioning, if ordered

  * Teach child and family that child should be placed on prophylactic antibiotic therapy prior to any dental work or surgical procedure (especially important with V-P shunt)

- **Emotional Care**

  * Promote growth and development

  * Provide support to family and child

  * Provide support group information to family

f. **Potential Complications** — Infection, obstruction or malfunction of shunt, subdural hematoma, infection or perforation of abdominal contents after placement. Death will occur if IICP is not detected or left untreated.

3. **NEURAL TUBE DEFECT**

   a. **Description** — The failure of the neural plate to close posteriorly in the midline. The most frequently seen defect is a myelomeningocele, a congenital defect where the spinal cord contents protrude through the spinal column in an enclosed sac-like structure. There are three major types: anencephaly (little or absent brain tissue; incompatible with life), encephalocele (midline defect in skull containing protruding cranial contents), myelodysplasia or spina bifida (malformation of vertebral column, meninges, and spinal cord).

b. **Signs and Symptoms** — Visual observation of defect; may have associated neurological defects such as loss of bladder and bowel control, and paraplegia. A less severe form of spina bifida (spina bifida occult) appears as a dimple on the lower sacral area but on further investigation it is noncystic and does not contain contents of the spinal cord.

c. **Diagnostic Procedures** — Diagnosed by physical findings, neurological exam determines level of defect; x-ray, MRI, CT scan, and ultrasound reveal spinal cord involvement and associated abnormalities such as hydrocephalus. Prenatal detection with ultrasound and elevated alpha-feto protein (AFP), amniocentesis.

d. **Medical Interventions**
   – **Medications** — Administer antibiotics (pre- and postoperatively), oxybutynin chloride (Ditropan), propantheline, stool softeners, laxatives, anticonvulsant, antispasmodics (for hypertonic bladder), choleric agents (for hypotonic bladder)
   – **Treatments** — Utilize correct positioning, maintain bowel and bladder care
   – **Surgery** — Surgical closure of defect is performed shortly after birth; continent ileal reservoir or urinary diversion may be necessary, V-P shunt if hydrocephalus

e. **Nursing Interventions**
   – **Assessment and Actions**
     * Assess newborn thoroughly for sign of defect
     * Protect sac covering preoperatively, keep sac moist with sterile gauze, place infant in heated environment, position infant in prone or side-lying position, avoid diapering; postoperatively: assess vital signs, hydration, level of comfort, nutrition, and place in prone or sidelying position, also monitor for increased intracranial pressure, signs of infection, place "donut" under head if V-P shunt placed to decrease pressure on shunt reservoir
     * Assess for signs indicating potential complications (infection, IICP, seizures)
     * Assess for latex allergy; use latex precautions and latex-free products
   – **Teaching**
     * Explain diagnosis to family and treatment regimen
     * Provide information regarding ROM exercises, positioning, mobilization devices, bladder and bowel elimination, and skin care; clean, intermittent catheterization (CIC)
     * Assist family with planning care for child once discharged
     * Use latex precautions to prevent latex allergy
   – **Emotional Care**
     * Promote child's growth and development
     * Provide support to family and child

* Provide support group information to family

f. **Potential Complications** — Disorder may also be accompanied by hydrocephalus, genitourinary disorders, paralysis, decubitus ulcers, dislocation of hips, delay in development, stress in family, bladder infections, meningitis, injury and infection of lower extremities, and latex allergy due to high risk in children who perform CIC.

Acquired Disorders

1. BACTERIAL MENINGITIS

   a. **Description** — An infection and inflammation of the meninges (coverings) of the brain usually due to *Hemophilus influenza* (type B), *Streptococcus pneumonia* or *Neisseria meningitidis*. Neonatal meningitis is most often caused by *E. coli* and group B streptococci. It may result from otitis media or sinusitis. It can be fatal.

   b. **Signs and Symptoms** — Depends upon organism, severity, and age of child; infants have vague and various signs and symptoms: bulging fontanel, headache, irritability, fever, seizure, drowsiness, poor feeding, vomiting, stiff neck, positive Kernig and Brudzinski signs, petechiae, apnea, jaundice, poor tone; children and adolescents: abrupt onset of fever, chills, headache, vomiting, altered neuro status, seizures, petechial or purpuric rash.

   c. **Diagnostic Procedures** — Diagnosed by positive lumbar puncture (LP), positive blood culture, elevated spinal fluid pressure and elevated WBC; if IICP suspected, CT scan may be ordered; if IICP confirmed, LP not performed to diminish risk of cranial herniation from sudden decrease in IICP.

   d. **Medical Interventions**
      – **Medications** — Administer antibiotic therapy appropriate for organism, anticonvulsant, antipyretics, electrolyte replacement, dexamethasone IV
      – **Treatments** — Monitor and relieve increased intracranial pressure and cerebral edema; monitor hydration and electrolyte status, and replace as necessary; isolation precautions
      – **Surgery** — Unnecessary

   e. **Nursing Interventions**
      – **Assessment and Action**
         * Maintain (Hib) immunizations up-to-date to prevent contraction of *H. influenzae*
         * Be alert for signs indicating disorder
         * Maintain medication therapy, hydration
         * Monitor neurological and respiratory status and provide quiet environment
         * Maintain respiratory body fluid isolation status
         * Provide method for reducing discomfort
         * Assess for signs indicating potential complications: change in V/S, LOC, urinary output

* Provide relief from fever with medications, tepid baths, cooling blanket
* Facilitate referral for rehabilitation services (hearing and speech), PT as needed

- **Teaching**

    * Explain procedures and treatment to family
    * Teach family importance of isolation and seizure control
    * Teach family about medications prescribed (drug, dose, route, time, and side effects)

- **Emotional Care**

    * Provide support to family and child
    * Provide support group information

f. **Potential Complications** — If treated promptly, uncommon; may experience disseminated intravascular coagulation (DIC) syndrome of inappropriate antidiuretic hormone secretion (SIADH), hearing impairment, hydrocephalus, peripheral circulatory collapse, permanent neurological impairment, meningococcemia (septic shock), death

2. ENCEPHALITIS

a. **Description** — An inflammation or infection of the brain resulting in swelling, cellular damage and temporary or permanent neurological dysfunction. It is most commonly caused by viral agents but may be bacterial or fungal in origin or result from toxins such as arsenic or lead. Majority of cases of known etiology are caused by childhood diseases such as chickenpox, measles, mumps, rubella, or herpes viruses.

b. **Signs and Symptoms** — Headache, lethargy, drowsiness, disturbance in speech, language, motor skills; seizures, change in level of consciousness, malaise, fever, dizziness, stiffness of neck, nausea, vomiting; onset may be gradual or rapid depending on cause.

c. **Diagnostic Procedures** — Diagnosed by physical findings, positive culture from lumbar puncture and Gram stain, brain biopsy, serologic antibody tests and MRI for brain hemorrhages.

d. **Medical Interventions**

- **Medications** — Administer antibiotics according to causative agent, steroids, osmotic diuretics, electrolyte replacement, anticonvulsant, antidotes to identified toxins
- **Treatment** — Supportive care and monitoring for complications
- **Surgery** — Unnecessary

e. **Nursing Interventions**

- **Assessment and Actions**

    * Monitor neuro status, vital signs, and provide comfort measures (dim lights, limit noise)
    * Facilitate appropriate referrals as necessary (speech therapy, OT, PT)

* Assess for signs indicating potential complications (seizures, permanent neuro impairment, death)

– **Teaching**

* Assess parents' level of understanding
* Discuss with parents and child procedures and treatment regimen allowing for questions
* Prepare parents and child for home care
* Teach parents about medication prescribed (drug, dose, route, time, and side effects)

– **Emotional Care**

* Encourage parents to visit child or remain with child while hospitalized
* Discuss the impact the neurological deficits, if present, have on parent and child
* Provide support to parents and child
* Provide support group information to family

  f. **Potential Complications** — Residual neurological deficits, delay in meeting developmental tasks, death.

3. **REYE'S SYNDROME**

  a. **Description** — A toxic invasion of the brain accompanied by severe cerebral edema, liver enlargement and fatty infiltration. It most commonly follows a viral infection and has been associated with the ingestion of aspirin. It most commonly occurs in males and has a high mortality rate.

  b. **Signs and Symptoms** — Initially has signs similar to common cold, then child appears to be well, followed by vomiting, hyperpnea, irregular respirations, dilated sluggish pupil reaction, and nervous system dysfunctions; neurological signs continue to progress from disorientation to various stages of coma; liver dysfunction and unresponsiveness follow.

  c. **Diagnostic Procedures** — Diagnosed by history of prodromal respiratory infection, influenza A or B, or chickenpox; presence of elevated AST (formerly SGOT) and ALT (formerly SGPT), LDH, bilirubin, and PTT; decreased serum glucose in children less than 5 years and hyperglycemia and pancreatitis in older children; abnormalities in EEG, increased serum ammonia, liver biopsy provides definite diagnosis.

  d. **Medical Interventions**

– **Medications** — Administer mannitol, insulin, vitamin K for clotting disturbances, anticonvulsant, and possibly barbiturates

– **Treatments** — Treatment depends upon stage of illness but includes:
Stage 1 — Maintain serum glucose level and reduce cerebral edema via IV fluids

Stages 2-5 — Reduce IICP, mannitol administration, tracheal intubation to control blood pH

– **Surgery** — Unnecessary

e. **Nursing Interventions**

– **Assessment and Actions**

* Be alert to signs and symptoms

* Monitor vital signs, IICP, cerebral edema, fluid status

* Assess for signs indicating potential complications

– **Teaching**

* Provide information on prevention of disorder including discouraging parents from utilizing aspirin and aspirin-containing products such as Pepto-Bismol™ during a child's illness

* Discuss with parents diagnosis, treatments, and allow parents to ask questions

– **Emotional Care**

* Provide support to family and child

* Provide support group information to family

f. **Potential Complications** — Neurological deficits, aspiration pneumonitis, respiratory failure, death.

4. **SEIZURE DISORDERS**

a. **Description** — Seizures are transient alterations in brain functioning resulting from overproduction of disorganized electrical charges and are manifested as alterations in level of consciousness or motor, sensory or autonomic functioning. They may be due to either congenital or acquired defects. They are categorized according to the cause and location of the neuronal discharge. Most seizures are idiopathic in nature.

b. **Signs and Symptoms** — Depend upon site of abnormal neurological discharge:

– **Categories Include:**

* **Partial seizures** — One hemisphere of the brain is usually affected:

   ° Complex partial seizures: Psychomotor seizures in which motor movement occurs without child's awareness (smacking, speaking, repetitive movement), child is amnesic of events, usually preceded by odor, taste, or sensation ("aura") and followed by sleep episode and postictal symptoms

   ° Simple partial seizures: Involuntary autonomic, sensory or motor function with child usually remaining conscious; various sensations including paresthesis, auras, pallor sweating

* **Generalized seizures** — Both hemispheres of the brain are affected:

  ° Absence seizures — Traditionally known as petit mal seizures; lapse in consciousness without associated movement; often seizure is unnoticed, may be mistaken for daydreaming

  ° Atonic and akinetic seizures — Inability to maintain posture and inability to move; sudden uncontrollable drop attacks with brief loss of consciousness

  ° Infantile spasms — Assumes flexed neck, drawn up legs and extended arms posture without loss of consciousness; often followed by crying or cooing (3 - 12 months typical age); disappears with age and often replaced by other type of seizure; associated with brain abnormality

  ° Myoclonic seizures — Muscle contraction followed by relaxation (single muscle group); child remains conscious

  ° Tonic clonic seizures — Traditionally known as grand mal seizures; contraction of muscles followed by jerking movement and relaxation: often exhibits cyanosis during contraction phase, bowel and bladder incontinence; child is unconscious during seizure

* **Other**

  ° Febrile seizure — Tonic clonic seizure due to extreme rise (usually >102°F or 39°C) in temperature, usually occurs only once during febrile episode, if fever brought under control it usually is without lasting effects

  ° Status epilepticus — Repetitive tonic clonic seizure without regaining consciousness between episodes; emergency — respiratory failure and death can ensue

c. **Diagnostic Procedures** — Diagnosed by identifying cause and may include: CBC, lumbar puncture, x-ray, CT scan; screening for TORCH (T-Toxoplasmosis, O-Other [such as hepatitis], R-Rubella, C-Cytomegalovirus, H-Herpes simplex); video monitored EEG to identify behavior associated with seizure, brain mapping

d. **Medical Interventions**

   – **Medications** — Administer anticonvulsant; e.g., carbamazepine, clonazepam, valporic acid, ethosuxamide, felbamate, phenobarbitol, phenytoin, primidone, lorazepam

   – **Treatments** — Treatment depends upon cause and type of seizure but requires anticonvulsant therapy and providing safety for child

   – **Surgery** — Surgical interventions may be necessary to diminish or eliminate the uncontrolled neuronal firing

e. **Nursing Interventions**

   – **Assessment and Actions**

   * Obtain detailed and thorough history

   * Be alert to signs and symptoms that indicate seizure disorder

* Assess seizure and monitor if certain events precede or follow
* Document seizures (onset, duration, pattern of movements, recovery)
* Maintain safe environment and utilize precautions
* Assess vital signs and neurological status of child
* Record serum level of anticonvulsant and monitor for side effects of medication
* Assess for signs indicating potential complications

– **Teaching**

* Teach parents and child about disorder, its cause and about treatment regimen; allow questions and explain on a level that a child can understand
* Inform parents about importance of seizure precautions and how to assist child during seizures (assist to floor, do not restrain, monitor breathing, do not force something into mouth, protect from injury, remove tight clothing, comfort child afterwards)
* Teach parents about medication prescribed (drug, dose, route, time, and side effects)
* Teach parents to use protective equipment (bike helmet) as needed
* Teach necessity of returning for follow-up visits/care and for drug level testing
* Stress importance of good dental hygiene if taking phenytoin

– **Emotional Care**

* Determine parents' and child's level of coping with disorder
* Assess anxiety level of parents and child
* Promote growth and development and enhance child's self-esteem
* Provide support to family and child
* Provide support group information to family

f. **Potential Complications** — Injury during seizures; numerous side effects from medications (behavior changes, bleeding problems, liver and kidney changes); possible drug toxicity; death (if respiratory failure occurs).

Sensory Disorders

1. **AUDITORY DISTURBANCES**

a. **Description** — The temporary or permanent loss of conductive, central auditory, sensorineural, or mixed sensorineural hearing. Hearing deficits are one of most common disabilities in childhood and range from slight to extreme hearing loss. Hearing loss can be congenital or acquired.

b. **Signs and Symptoms** — Vary; may find a diminished startle reflex and low score for response to human voice on Brazelton Neonatal Assessment in neonates; difficulty in learning, speech delay or delay in response to voice; increased visual attention, diminished response to verbal directions; behavior problems or withdrawn behavior.

c. **Diagnostic Procedures** — Audiometry reveals diminished or absent hearing, tympanometry reveals decreased movement, brainstem auditory evoked potentials show decreased brain potential.

d. **Medical Interventions**
   - **Medications** — Administer antibiotics if infection is present
   - **Treatments** — Treatment depends on cause and severity of loss, but ranges from hearing aids to surgical implants or corrections
   - **Surgery** — May require surgical implant or tube placement

e. **Nursing Interventions**
   - **Assessment and Actions**
     * Be alert for signs and symptoms that indicate a hearing loss
     * Prevent by keeping child's immunizations current, monitoring or reducing loud noises in the environment, appropriately treating otitis media
     * Notify school nurse/teachers, other parents, and friends of deficit and how to communicate
     * Facilitate referral (speech therapy, audiology)
     * Assess for signs indicating potential complications
   - **Teaching**
     * Explain to parent and child significance and duration of loss
     * Provide information on diagnosis, treatment and methods of coping with deficit: use of hearing aid, sign language, lip reading, speech therapy, ways to enhance child's growth and development
   - **Emotional Care**
     * Promote growth and development and socialization
     * Provide support to family and child
     * Provide support group information to family

f. **Potential Complications** — Potential for delay in development and socialization.

2. VISUAL DISTURBANCES

a. **Description** — Any alteration in vision. It may be due to a variety of factors and may be congenital (cataracts, glaucoma), or acquired (trauma, Retinopathy of Prematurity [ROP], retinoblastoma). The disturbance may be categorized as an acute or chronic disorder. It may range from slight impairment to complete impairment.

b. **Signs and Symptoms** — Depend on type and severity; may have poor motor control of eyes (strabismus), diminished vision in one eye (amblyopia), visual opaqueness in lens (cataract), increased intraocular pressure (glaucoma), visible wound or abnormality of eye (trauma or malformation), inability to make eye contact or follow objects, may not reach for items, may bump into things, or complain of inability to see, may show a delay in fine and gross motor skills as development continues, may exhibit poor school work, frequently rub eyes or squint, exhibit poor peripheral vision.

c. **Diagnostic Procedures** — Diagnosed by finding abnormalities in the following tests: Neonatal Brazelton Assessment Scoring, visual assessment with and without ophthalmoscope, funduscopic examination, vision screening (Snellen chart), slit lamp exam.

d. **Medical Interventions**

- **Medications** — May require miotic therapy or antibiotics (if infection present)
- **Treatments** — Depend on cause and severity of visual disturbance; may require correction with lenses or patching of eye
- **Surgery** — Corrective surgery may be necessary for persistent strabismus, cataracts, glaucoma, or foreign body removal

e. **Nursing Interventions**

- **Assessment and Actions**
  * Screen children at early age and detect abnormalities
  * Monitor child's ability to perform ADLs
  * Provide safe environment if hospitalized
  * Familiarize child with environment
  * Introduce self and speak to child when entering or exiting room
  * Assess for signs indicating potential complications

- **Teaching**
  * Provide anticipatory guidance by making parent and child aware of safety needs of eyes
  * Explain findings of eye exam to parent and child
  * Provide education for parents according to necessary treatment: necessity of glasses or lenses and proper care, instillation of eye drops (drug, dose, times, and side effects), care of prosthesis
  * Prepare child and family for surgical correction as appropriate and what to expect before, during and after surgery
  * Teach parents how to interact with child if impairment is severe and permanent; familiarize child with environment and don't change it suddenly; promote bonding; enhance development; encourage independence; provide safety for child; assist with schooling and inform teachers of child's special needs; use braille, assistive devices

- **Emotional Care**
  * Discuss impact diagnosis has on child and family
  * Promote growth, development and socialization
  * Provide support to family and child

* Provide support group information to family

f. **Potential Complications** — Delay in growth and development, post-operative infection, injury due to visual deficit.

Disorders Arising from Trauma

1. **COMA**

   a. **Description** — A temporary or permanent alteration in alertness or consciousness in which the child is not aroused with even strong stimulus. It may include: unresponsiveness to specific stimuli, absence of reflexes, lack of spontaneous breathing, and flat EEG. It may be the result of a variety of cerebral insults and may be categorized from light coma to brain death.

   b. **Signs and Symptoms** — Altered or abnormal neurological scoring in relation to eye opening, motor and verbal response using a pediatric coma scale or Glasgow Coma scale.

   c. **Diagnostic Procedures** — Diagnosed by physical findings; diagnosis procedures utilized depend on causative factor but may include culture and sensitivity to rule out organisms; evaluation of blood oxygen levels to rule out hypoxia; lumbar puncture to rule out organisms and cancerous diagnosis, EEG to determine brain activity; and CT scan to determine if mass is present; urinalysis or serology to determine if toxin present or if metabolic cause.

   d. **Medical Interventions**
      - **Medications** — Medications given according to causative factor or to treat possible complications and may include corticosteroids, barbiturates, diuretics
      - **Treatments** — Maintain vital functions, monitor ICP and neurological status, monitor for and treat complications
      - **Surgery** — May be necessary if due to pressure or mass in brain

   e. **Nursing Interventions**
      - **Assessment and Actions**
        * Assess child's neurological status as ordered, noting changes
        * Monitor vital signs, respiratory status, hydration, nutrition, bowel and bladder functioning, and skin temperature and intactness
        * Document neuro status as ordered
        * Assess for signs indicating potential complications
        * If appropriate discuss brain death and potential organ donation
      - **Teaching**
        * Discuss diagnosis and treatment regimen with parents, allowing for questions
        * Provide information regarding safety of child to prevent head injuries, near drownings, or other trauma that may lead to neurological insults leading to comatose state

* Teach parents how to care for child (feeding, bathing, exercising, turning)
  - **Emotional Care**
    * Speak to child during procedures
    * Provide support to parents and assess coping level
    * Provide support group information to parents
  f. **Potential Complications** — Skin breakdown, contractures (if long-term) respiratory or bladder infections, residual neurological damage, and death

2. **HEAD INJURY**

   a. **Description** — An open or closed injury to the cranium and its contents resulting from mechanical force. The term head injury includes concussions, contusions, skull fractures, vascular injuries, and cerebral edema. The prognosis depends on the extent of the injury.

   b. **Signs and Symptoms** — Depend on severity but include: headache, loss of consciousness, bradycardia, hypotension, CSF leakage from an orifice, vomiting, irritability, increased intracranial pressure, seizures, increased sleepiness, behavioral disturbances.

   c. **Diagnostic Procedures** — Diagnosed by physical findings; diagnostic tests utilized depend on history of injury but may include the following: skull x-ray may show damage, EEG may exhibit alteration, CT scan may show bleeding, cerebral angiography reveals hemorrhaging.

   d. **Medical Interventions**
      - **Medications** — Administer antibiotics if open injury present; may require osmotic diuretics if cerebral swelling present; may administer anticonvulsants
      - **Treatments** — Depend on severity of injury but may include home observation, monitoring airway, treating for shock, aspiration of fluid, monitoring of vital signs and ICP
      - **Surgery** — Surgical intervention may be necessary if hemorrhaging is present or cranium is fractured or crushed

   e. **Nursing Interventions**
      - **Assessment and Actions**
        * Always assume child has cervical and spinal injuries until ruled out
        * Be alert to signs and symptoms that may indicate injury
        * Maintain airway and stabilize head and neck
        * Obtain a careful history if head injury suspected
        * Assess vital signs and level of consciousness frequently
        * Be alert for signs of contrecoup injuries (signs of internal injury on the side opposite the direct injury to the head)

* If hospitalization is required, monitor vital signs, neuro status, including reflexes and level of consciousness, maintain bedrest, keep environment quiet, assess for any drainage from ears or nose, periorbital ecchymosis (raccoon eyes), postauricular ecchymosis (Battle sign), observe for signs of increased intracranial pressure, assess for other injuries, provide only clear liquids until stable and alert
* Assess for signs of non-accidental trauma (NAT), and shaken baby syndrome
* Assess for signs indicating potential complications
* Report injury if child abuse suspected; facilitate social services interventions
* Facilitate rehabilitative services as needed (PT, OT)

   – **Teaching**

* Provide anticipatory guidance to parents by informing them of the higher risk of head injuries in children and suggest ways to diminish injury
* Discuss with parents diagnoses and treatment regimen, if home care needed, teach parents to observe for abnormal signs and symptoms (change in level of consciousness and/or in pupils, presence of double vision, change in coordination) and when to contact the physician

   – **Emotional Care**

* Provide support to family and child
* Provide support group information to family

  f. **Potential Complications** — Infection, neurological deficits, coma, death.

3. **INCREASED INTRACRANIAL PRESSURE**

  a. **Description** — An increase in the normal pressure of the CSF. It may be caused by excess production of CSF, obstruction of flow of CSF, or increased size of brain mass (due to swelling, injury, infection or tumors).

  b. **Signs and Symptoms** — Depend upon age; infants (before suture lines close): enlarged head circumference, bulging fontanels, setting sun eyes, high-pitched cry, poor feeding; children: headache, vomiting, irritability, change in level of consciousness, drowsiness, poor attention span; as pressure increases signs may include: change in vital signs, loss of consciousness, change in pupils, altered or clumsy movements; change in posturing (decerebrate or decorticate posture), seizures, respiratory arrest.

  c. **Diagnostic Procedures** — Diagnosed by physical findings, CSF reveals increased pressure; CT scan and MRI reveal mass or blockage; EEG may reveal decreased activity.

d. **Medical Interventions**

- **Medications** — Administer osmotic diuretics (Mannitol), restrict fluids, and administer steroids, barbiturates, antacids, cimetidime or ranitidime, antipyretics
- **Treatments** — Monitor vital signs, respiratory and neurological status, IICP monitoring by subarachnoid bolt, hyperventilation (to decrease $PaCO_2$ and increase PaO_2 thereby decreasing cerebral edema)
- **Surgery** — Surgical correction by removal of mass, stopping hemorrhaging, or opening passageway for flow of CSF production, V-P or V-A shunt placement, extraventricular drain (EVD) placement

e. **Nursing Interventions**

- **Assessment and Actions**
  * Be alert to signs of IICP
  * Monitor IICP, VS, respiratory functioning, neuro status (including subtle changes in level of consciousness, personality, and motor function); elevate head of bed 30-45 degrees and keep head in neutral alignment, avoid flexion of neck; keep environment quiet
  * Monitor fluid status and nutrition
  * Administer medications as ordered
  * Assess for signs indicating potential complications

- **Teaching**
  * Explain to family diagnosis and treatment regimen
  * Teach parents about medication prescribed (drug, dose, route, time and side effects)

- **Emotional Care**
  * Provide support to family and child
  * Provide support group information to family

f. **Potential Complications** — Infection, neurological deficits, respiratory failure, death.

Other

1. **ATTENTION DEFICIT HYPERACTIVITY DISORDER (ADHD)**

a. **Description** — The inability to control attention span, impulses, and activity level appropriate for age. It is a type of learning disability of unknown etiology. It is more commonly seen in males. It appears to be a genetic component, as well as associated with maternal alcohol abuse and metabolic and/or infectious diseases during childhood.

b. **Signs and Symptoms** — Depend on severity but may include inability to maintain attention level, exhibition of hyperactivity, inability to delay impulses, easily frustrated, inability to complete a task, highly distractable, poor social skills; symptoms usually present before 7 years of age and have lasted at least 6 months.

c. **Diagnostic Procedures** — Diagnosed by reviewing history and descriptive report by parents and teachers, utilizing psychological screening; EEG may reveal abnormal findings; CT scan may show mild cerebral atrophy; vision and hearing evaluations to rule out sensory abnormality; serology to rule out lead poisoning.

d. **Medical Interventions**
   – **Medications** — Administer methylphenidate, dextroamphetamine, or pemoline (Ritalin, Dexedrine or Silar)
   – **Treatment** — May require psychotherapy or behavior modification
   – **Surgery** — Unnecessary

e. **Nursing Interventions**
   – **Assessment and Actions**
      * Be alert to signs and symptoms of ADHD
      * Network with school nurse and teachers
      * Monitor factors causing exacerbations (foods, environment, time of day)
      * Facilitate appropriate referral (behavior therapist)
      * Assess for signs indicating potential complications
   – **Teaching**
      * Explain disorder and treatment regimen to parents and child
      * Discuss medication therapy and potential side effects
      * Assist parent with behavior therapy and reducing environmental stimulation
   – **Emotional Care**
      * Discuss impact disorder has on child and family
      * Promote growth and development, as well as healthy social interaction
      * Provide support to family and child
      * Provide support group information to family

f. **Potential Complications** — Medication side effects may produce growth retardation or delay in developmental level or toxicity: cardiac arrhythmias, thrombocytopenia; developmental delay may be prevented by decreasing the dose of the medication or stopping the medication periodically.

12

ONCOLOGY DISORDERS

I. General Concepts

- Cancer is defined as the occurrence and overproduction of abnormal cells

- Cancer may develop in any tissue

- The cause of cancer is unknown but may be related to genetics, the environment, and nutritional intake

- Cancer is categorized according to its level of development and sites where metastasis has occurred

- Cardinal signs and symptoms of most cancers include: pain, anorexia, fatigue, weight loss, change in behavior, frequent infection, bleeding episodes, fever, and open sore(s) that will not heal

- Cancer is considered to be cured if the tumor does not occur within five years of completing treatment

II. Specific Treatments

* Regimens for malignant tumors typically follow specific protocols for the particular cancerous cells but may include the following:

Bone Marrow Transplants

The placement of healthy bone marrow into a diseased area. It may be retrieved from an allogenic (related or unrelated donor), autologous (donor and recipient are the same), or a syngeneic donor (donor and recipient are identical twins). Additional sources include peripheral blood stem cells (autologous) and fetal cord blood. It requires long-term hospitalization, immunosuppression prior to and after transplantation and isolation. Complications include infection and graft vs. host disease (GVHD).

Chemotherapy

The administration of antineoplastic agents*. It may be used as the only treatment or may be combined with other therapies. The placement of a long-term catheter for drug administration is required (Port or Broviac). Chemotherapy is classified according to the action of the drug and may include the use of the following categories:

1. **Alkylating Agents**: Chlorambucil, Cyclophosphamide, busulfan, ifosfamide, procarbazine, dacarbazine, Mechlorethamine

2. **Antibiotics:** Actinomycin-D, Bleomycin, Daunorubicin, and Doxorubicin, mitomycin, idarubicin, mitoxantrone

3. **Antimetabolites:** 5-Azacytidine, Cytosine arabinoside, Mercaptopurine, Methotrexate, and 6-Thioguanine, 5-fluorouracil

4. **Enzymes:** L-asparaginases

5. **Hormones:** Corticosteroids

6. **Plant Alkaloids**: Vincristine and Vinblastine, VP-16 etoposide, VM teniposide

7. **Others**: Cisplatin, carboplatin, Dacarbazine, Hydroxyurea, and Procarbazine

8. **Nitrosoureas:** carmustine, homustine

9. **Biologic Response Modifiers:** IL-1, IL-2, interferon

---

* Each agent has specific side effects. The most commonly seen reactions include nausea, vomiting, anorexia, alopecia, stomatitis, diarrhea, abdominal pain, dermatitis, weight loss. Extremely high doses may affect the heart and nervous system.

Biologic Response Modifiers (BRMs)

Modify the relationship between tumor and host by therapeutically changing the host's biologic response to tumor cells. Interventions can have direct antitumor activity, affect the immunologic mechanisms (immunotherapy), or have other biologic effects.

Palliative Therapy

Treatments which provide comfort and relieve pain or pressure. These treatments are not intended to cure. It includes the reduction of side effects of medication or treatments, the surgical removal of the tumor to decrease discomfort, and the administration of analgesics or narcotics.

Radiotherapy

The administration of ionizing radiation to the diseased area. The side effects depend upon the location that is being treated but include nausea, vomiting, diarrhea, GI ulceration, alopecia, dermatitis, cystitis, and anemia. In situations where unresectable residual disease remains due to proximity of vital structures or unavoidable rupture of the tumor, intraoperative radiation to the tumor bed can be utilized.

Surgical Removal

The excision of all or part of the diseased area. It may be a curative or palliative procedure or assist in slowing the growth process of the tumor.

III. General Nursing Interventions

Assessment and Actions

1. Be alert to signs and symptoms of cancer.

2. Diminish potential for infection by maintaining isolation.

3. Monitor vital signs and I&O during drug administration.

4. Assess infusion site carefully for signs of extravasation and stop infusion and notify MD immediately if infiltration occurs.

5. Promote nutrition by offering foods requested, small meals, mild-flavored food; avoid offering favorite foods during periods of nausea; provide mouth care, and decrease offensive odors in room or environment; administering antiemetics before meals and before/during chemotherapy administration may also help; apply anesthetics to ulcers in mouth and monitor weight daily.

6. Encourage activity as tolerated, including rest periods each day.

7. Provide therapy for potential neuropathies as they occur (foot drop, jaw pain, difficulty walking) and report findings — may indicate need for dose adjustment.

8. Provide for comfort by repositioning, using gentle massage, warmth, cold application, analgesic administration, relaxation.

9. Assess for signs indicating potential complications (specific to medications or location of tumor).

10. Maintain a clean environment.

11. Monitor hemotologic parameters — hgb, plt ct, WBC/Neutrophil count.

Teaching

1. Prepare child and family for diagnostic procedures by explaining type of procedure and preparations that are necessary before and after procedure.

2. Explain diagnosis and discuss treatment regimen.

3. Assess family and child's level of understanding.

4. Instruct family and child on methods for reducing discomfort.

5. Instruct family and child on importance of preventing exposure of child to infection.

6. Teach family and child care of central line.

7. Teach family and child how to select foods which will increase protein intake and to avoid foods which may cause nausea.

8. Prepare child and family for procedures and treatments by providing appropriate information on what to expect before, during, and after each necessary activity (bone marrow aspiration, lumbar puncture, medication administration, port or catheter placement).

9. Teach parents and child about medication prescribed (drug, dose, route, and side effects).

10. Discuss long-term care needs as appropriate.

11. Teach family and child to recognize signs/symptoms which may indicate a serious condition (infection, fever, neutropenia, bleeding, etc.)

12. Prepare parents and child for discharge.

13. Teach parents and child to prevent contact with others who are sick while immunocompromised.

Emotional Care

1. Promote child's growth and development while being treated by enhancing independence with activities appropriate for age.

2. Provide family with an environment which allows questions and concerns to be considered and answered.

3. Discuss with child and family how disease is impacting lifestyle.

4. Discuss with child how he is adapting to change in body image.

5. Assist child with adapting to loss of body part or change in body appearance.

6. Provide honest information, do not give false reassurance.

7. Be prepared to discuss death with parent or child and listen to concerns or beliefs.

8. Provide emotional support to family and child.

9. Provide support group information to family and child.

10. Allow for grieving and anger, assure child and family that this is part of the grieving process.

11. Encourage parents to provide opportunities for siblings to express needs and feelings openly without judgment.

IV. Specific Oncology Disorders

1. BRAIN TUMORS

a. **Description** — Abnormal tissue growth within the cranium. It may be infratentorial or supratentorial in location. It is categorized according to the tissue that is affected. The most common brain tumors in the pediatric population are astrocytomas. The survival rate for brain tumors ranges from 25% to 90% depending upon the location and response of the tumor to treatment.

b. **Signs and Symptoms** — Depend upon age of child, anatomical location and size of tumor; child may not exhibit signs until late in disease process if suture lines of skull are not closed; findings include headache and vomiting especially after arising in the morning, dizziness, irritability, drowsiness, change in motor control, weakness, failure to thrive, change in level of consciousness or behavior, altered vision, change in vital signs, seizures, nuchal rigidity.

c. **Diagnostic Procedures** — Diagnosed by reviewing history and abnormal physical findings especially in neurological status; CT scan allows for visualization of mass, angiography shows vascular supply to tumor, MRI reveals location and size of mass, intracranial biopsy determines whether mass is benign or malignant.

d. **Medical Interventions**
   – **Medications** — Administer chemotherapy according to specific protocol

– **Treatments** — Administer radiation therapy

– **Surgery** — Surgical excision of tumor if possible

– **Bone Marrow Transplant**

e. **Nursing Interventions** — (See previous list of General Nursing Interventions)

   – **Assessment and Actions**
   * Preoperatively monitor child's vital signs and neuro status
   * Postoperatively monitor vital signs, fluid status, neuro status; position patient with head in midline and elevate head of bed as ordered; keep environment as quiet as possible; provide method for reducing discomfort

   – **Teaching**
   * Prepare child and family for treatment regimen by describing what to expect before, during, and after surgical procedure
   * Explain side effects of chemotherapy and radiation therapy and how to reduce side effects
   * Discuss long-term therapy that is necessary after discharge

   – **Emotional Care**
   * Do not provide false hope and be honest with family and child
   * Encourage family to continue routine life at home as much as possible
   * Provide suggestions for alternatives for covering head after surgery to promote child's body image

f. **Potential Complications** - Neurological impairment (paralysis, visual or auditory impairment, coma, seizures — depends on area of brain affected or removed), infection, delays in growth and development, and death.

2. **EWING'S SARCOMA**

   a. **Description** — A tumor of the bone and/or soft tissues (peripheral neuroectodermal tumor [PNET]). It usually affects the long bones and bones of the trunk. It is a highly malignant tumor.

   b. **Signs and Symptoms** — Bone pain and discomfort, swelling in affected area.

   c. **Diagnostic Procedures** — Diagnosed by physical findings, bone marrow aspiration reveals abnormal cells, x-ray reveals bone destruction, and surgical biopsy confirms diagnosis and whether tumor is benign or malignant.

   d. **Medical Interventions**

      – **Medications** — Administer chemotherapy according to specific protocol
      – **Treatment** — Administer radiation therapy to area
      – **Surgery** — Surgical amputation is not routinely recommended but may be considered

    e. **Nursing Interventions** — (See previous list of General Nursing Interventions)

        – **Assessment and Actions**

          * Preoperatively monitor vital signs and provide methods for reducing discomfort

          * Postoperatively monitor vital signs, site for hemorrhaging, elevate amputation above level of the heart, monitor I&O, and provide method for reducing pain (administer analgesics, anti-inflammatous, narcotics as ordered)

          * Assist with returning child to ambulatory status as soon as possible

        – **Teaching**

          * Explain effects of treatment and ways to relieve discomfort

          * Explain that use of extremity need not be limited

          * Prepare family and child for long-term treatment regimen

          * If surgical resection or amputation is necessary, explain treatment, allow for questions and concerns to be addressed

          * Teach crutch-walking and placement and use of prosthesis as necessary

        – **Emotional Care**

          * Promote return to normal lifestyle as soon as possible

          * Support family and child during time of grieving

          * Discuss with child the impact disorder has had on lifestyle and body image

    f. **Potential Complications** — Bone fragility, infection, death.

3. **LEUKEMIA**

    a. **Description** — A primary malignancy of the bone marrow and lymphatic system which causes overproduction of immature WBCs. The most commonly seen types of leukemia are acute lymphocytic leukemia (80% are ALL) and acute myelogenous (nonlymphocytic) leukemia (AML or ANL). The prognosis of leukemia depends upon differentiation (ALL generally more favorable), cytogenetic evaluation, and cell surface markers.

    b. **Signs and Symptoms** — Anemia, pallor, fractures, fever, bone pain, fatigue, lassitude, anorexia, frequent infections, bleeding episodes, petechiae, lymphadenopathy, hepatosplenomegaly, hyperuremia.

    c. **Diagnostic Procedures** — Diagnosed by history of signs and symptoms: blood smears reveal immature WBC; CBC reveals anemia, neutropenia, thrombocytopenia; lumbar puncture reveals evidence of CMS disease; bone marrow aspiration is the definitive diagnostic test.

    d. **Medical Interventions**

        – **Medications** — Attempt to induce remission by use of chemotherapy according to specific protocol followed by CNS prophylaxis (intrathecal chemotherapy) and maintenance therapy for 30-36 months

- **Treatments** — Administer radiation therapy in high risk patients
- **Bone Marrow Transplantation**

e. **Nursing Interventions** — (See previous list of General Nursing Interventions)

  - **Assessment and Actions**
    * While hospitalized monitor V/S, nutritional intake, I&O, bleeding episodes, level of activity tolerance, and level of comfort
    * Discuss life threatening potential of contracting chickenpox and need for prompt treatment if thought to be exposed
    * Discuss need for platelet transfusion and frequency
    * Provide antiemetic medication to prevent or diminish nausea
  - **Teaching**
    * Emphasize prevention of infection and prompt treatment of minor injuries (neutropenic precautions, possibly wearing helmet to protect brain, avoidance of dangerous activities such as diving)
    * Explain procedures, treatment regimen and side effects of medications
    * Explain need to prevent injury to any area, utilize soft toothbrush or toothettes
    * Explain importance of maintaining nutrition and fluid intake
    * Teach parents signs and symptoms which require MD to be notified (fever, bleeding, pain, extreme fatigue, infection); reassure that, in time, the family will return to a "routine"
  - **Emotional Care**
    * Discuss impact disease has on family and child

f. **Potential Complications** — Infections, relapse, bleeding.

4. **HODGKIN'S DISEASE**

  a. **Description** — A malignant growth of the lymphoid system. It often metastasizes to other organs such as the liver, bone marrow, spleen, and lungs. It is treated according to the classification and stage of the neoplasm: stages I-IV. It affects adolescents more frequently than younger age groups and males more than females. It has a good prognosis.

  b. **Signs and Symptoms** — Enlarged, non-tender, moveable lymph nodes typically in cervical area; fever, nausea, vomiting, weight loss, cough, night sweats, generalized pruritus, splenomegaly; other symptoms depend upon areas of metastasis.

  c. **Diagnostic Procedures** — Diagnosed by history and physical; CBC reveals neutrophilia, eosinophilia, lymphocytopenia; CT; biopsy reveals abnormal cells.

d. **Medical Interventions**

- **Medications** — Administer chemotherapy according to specific protocol
- **Treatments** — Administer radiation therapy
- **Surgery** — May require surgical removal of tumors that have metastasized, may require splenectomy and laparotomy

e. **Nursing Interventions** — (See previous list of General Nursing Interventions)

- **Assessment and Actions**
  * Be alert for signs and symptoms
  * Discuss diagnosis treatment with family
  * Monitor for side effects of chemotherapy
  * Preoperatively provide comfort measures and monitor vital signs
  * Postoperatively monitor vital signs, level of comfort, incision, bowel sounds, and for signs of infection
  * Be alert to signs indicating potential complications
- **Teaching**
  * Instruct family and child on methods to reduce side effects of treatment
  * Prepare child and family for treatment regimen by describing what to expect before and during and after surgical procedure
- **Emotional Care**
  * Discuss how diagnosis and treatment regimen have impacted child's and family's life

f. **Potential Complications** — Infections, pulmonary emboli from lymphangiography, delayed secondary sexual development, retardation of bone growth and soft tissue development, especially in younger children; death if widespread metastasis present.

5. **NEUROBLASTOMAS**

a. **Description** — Tumors which develop from the embryonic neural crest cells. They typically affect the adrenal gland and peritoneal structures. They are classified and treated according to staging (I-IV). They have a poor prognosis in patients >12 months of age and/or within Stage III or IV disease.

b. **Signs and Symptoms** — Usually asymptomatic until after metastasis occurs; symptoms depend on site affected; typically palpable abdominal mass, change in voiding with frequency or retention, lymphadenopathy, periorbital edema and ecchymosis, heterochromia (irises of different colors); if ophthalmic sympathetic nerves involved, cardinal signs of cancer.

c. **Diagnostic Procedures** — Diagnosed by physical findings; CT scan identifies site(s); bone scan; gallium scan; abdominal ultrasound; clumped cancer cells on bone marrow aspiration; biopsy reveals abnormal cells, measurement of tumor markers — VMA, HVA, catecholamines, bone marrow aspirate.

d. **Medical Interventions**

 – **Medications** — Administer chemotherapy according to specific protocol

 – **Treatments** — Administer radiation therapy; dialysis is utilized if nephrectomy necessary

 – **Surgery** — Surgical removal of tumor(s) may be required (stages I-III), nephrectomy performed if kidney involved

 – **Bone Marrow Transplant**

e. **Nursing interventions** — (See previous list of General Nursing Interventions)

 – **Assessment and Actions**

 * Prevent palpation of mass after diagnosis is made

 * Preoperatively monitor vital signs and urine output

 * Postoperatively monitor vital signs, I&O, urine output, and provide method for reducing discomfort

 * Obtain a complete and accurate urine collection for markers

 – **Teaching**

 * Reinforce critical nature of diagnosis with parents and child if appropriate

 * Prepare child for dialysis if treatment warrants by explaining what to expect before, during, and after treatment

 – **Emotional Care**

 * Encourage child to maintain as routine a lifestyle as possible

 * Provide support to family during grieving period

f. **Potential Complications** — Infection, metastasis, death.

6. **NON-HODGKIN'S LYMPHOMA**

a. **Description** — A diffuse generalized malignancy of the lymphoid system. Its most common presentation is intra-abdominal and is often associated with meningeal and mediastinal involvement. It is more commonly seen in boys. Survival rates are 50-80% but treatment is palliative if relapse occurs.

b. **Signs and Symptoms** — Depend upon sites affected; lymphadenopathy, fatigue, anorexia, weight loss, night sweats, may exhibit signs of leukemia, abdominal pain and acute respiratory symptoms (mediastinal).

c. **Diagnostic Procedures** — Diagnosed by physical findings, biopsy reveals abnormal cells, bone marrow aspiration reveals abnormal cells, x-ray reveals location, and CT scan determines area affected.

d. **Medical Interventions**

 – **Medications** — Administer chemotherapy according to specific protocol

- **Treatments** — Administer radiation therapy
- **Surgery** — Surgical resection and excision may be performed in some cases

e. **Nursing Interventions** — (See previous list of General Nursing Interventions)

     - **Assessment and Actions**

         * Implement nursing care similar to treating the child with leukemia

         * Monitor patient's V/S, I&O, nutritional status

         * Assess level of discomfort and provide means for pain control

         * Monitor for tumor lysis syndrome

     - **Teaching**

         * Explain diagnosis and treatment plan

         * Teach importance of meeting nutritional requirements and means for meeting caloric intake

         * Teach parents about medications prescribed (drug, dose, route, time, and side effects)

     - **Emotional Care**

         * Discuss impact diagnosis has on family and child

         * Provide support during grieving period

f. **Potential Complications** — Infections, death, tumor lysis syndrome, bleeding, pulmonary obstruction.

7. **OSTEOGENIC SARCOMA (OSTEOSARCOMA)**

     a. **Description** — A malignancy affecting bone tissue (particularly long bones). It is the most commonly seen bone tumor in children. It frequently metastasizes to the lungs and is more common in males and may be related to adolescent growth spurts. It is rare before age 10 and is most common between 10 and 25.

     b. **Signs and Symptoms** — Dull aching or pain in bone, may exhibit limp or guarded extremity, decreased activity level, swelling or redness in area, other cardinal signs of cancer.

     c. **Diagnostic Procedures** — Diagnosed by considering history and physical assessment; CT scan and MRI are used to assess extent of disease prior to surgery; x-ray reveals sunburst or ray of needles in bone formation; biopsy necessary to confirm diagnosis.

     d. **Medical Interventions**

         - **Medications** — Administer chemotherapy according to specific protocol

         - **Treatments** — Radiation therapy is ineffective as tumor is radioresistant

         - **Surgery** — Surgical removal of bone/partial bone with prosthetic or cadaver graft (limb salvage) replacement, or amputation of extremity is performed

e. **Nursing Interventions** — (See previous list of General Nursing Interventions)

  – **Assessment and Actions**

  * Preoperatively provide pain control therapy

  * Postoperatively monitor vital signs, hemorrhaging status, elevate amputated extremity above the heart, monitor I&O, provide pain control

  * Provide stump care and be prepared for child to complain of phantom limb pain or sensations

  * Assist child with ambulation with prosthetic device as soon as possible to promote self-mobilization

  * Use of continuous motion device for limb salvage involving joint

  – **Teaching**

  * Discuss amputation and what will happen before, during, and after surgery/graft/prosthesis

  * Teach stump care to family and application of prosthesis

  * Teach family and child to protect newly-amputated area and be alert to signs of infection

  * Reinforce expectations of bone prosthesis (may not be able to walk without crutches, run, swim, or ride a bike)

  – **Emotional Care**

  * Prepare child and family for surgical resection or amputation

  * Provide support to family during grieving period

  * Provide time for child and family to discuss change in body image and identify ways that child can cope

  * Promote normal growth and development throughout treatment

  f. **Potential Complications** — Infection, lung metastasis, death.

8. **RETINOBLASTOMA**

  a. **Description** — A hereditary, malignant tumor of one or both retinas. It arises from transmission of a mutated, defective gene or spontaneous cell mutations. The prognosis depends upon the staging (Group 1 — best prognosis, Group 5 — poor prognosis). The symptoms usually occur before two years of age. Survival rate is good but may include loss of vision.

  b. **Signs and Symptoms** — White reflex in eye (appears as Cat's eye reflex on simple visual inspection) often accompanied by strabismus and change in visual acuity; may cause blindness in late stage.

  c. **Diagnostic Procedures** — Diagnosed by abnormal findings in ophthalmic examination during scleral indentation, fiberoptic transillumination, and tomograms of orbit; also presence of elevated LDH in aqueous humor; positive family history.

  d. **Medical Interventions**

  – **Medications** — Administer chemotherapy

- **Treatments** — Depends upon staging; staging 1-3 require radiation therapy; photocoagulation, cryotherapy, or radioactive applicators may be utilized
- **Surgery** — States 1-3 require cryotherapy and coagulation of specific retinal blood vessels; stages 4-5 often require surgical enucleation

e. **Nursing Interventions** — (See previous list of General Nursing Interventions)

- **Assessment and Actions**
  * Assess vision before and after treatment
  * Monitor for signs of infection postoperatively
  * Provide method of pain control
  * Provide safe environment and appropriate activities/stimulation for sight-impaired child
- **Teaching**
  * Teach parents care of and placement of prosthetic device and orbital socket
  * Assist parent and child in maintaining a safe environment and help child adapt to visual change and, if appropriate, loss of eye
  * Arrange genetic counseling
- **Emotional Care**
  * Prepare child and family for appearance after enucleation
  * Discuss impact on family and how family is coping

f. **Potential Complications** — Blindness, infection.

9. **RHABDOMYOSARCOMA**

a. **Description** — An aggressively malignant tumor of the soft tissue (muscles, connective tissue, lymphatic tissue, tendons, vascular tissue). It arises from embryonal tissue and may occur anywhere in the body where striated muscle is found. It occurs most often between 2 and 6 years. It is staged according to the sites and metastasis (Group 1-4). Forty percent occur in the head, orbit and neck, 35% in genitourinary and abdominal areas and 25% in the trunk and extremities. The prognosis is good if remission is achieved. If relapse occurs, survival rate is poor.

b. **Signs and Symptoms** — Depends upon site of tumor but most common signs are painless mass or functional impairment of affected site; may also include: visible mass, wound which does not heal, pain in area, swelling, frequent ear infections, lymphadenopathy; symptoms may not occur until tumor becomes enlarged and begins to put pressure on other tissues in the area.

c. **Diagnostic Procedures** — Diagnosed by direct inspection and palpation, x-ray and CT scans reveal location; bone marrow aspiration and lumbar puncture show abnormal cells; MRI shows location and size of tumor; tissue biopsy reveals abnormal cells.

d. **Medical Interventions**

  – **Medications** — Administer chemotherapy according to specific protocol

  – **Treatments** — Administer radiation therapy

  – **Surgery** — Surgical removal of tumor performed if tumor can be completely excised

e. **Nursing Interventions** — (See previous list of General Nursing Interventions)

  – **Assessment and Actions**

   * Provide method for pain control

   * Assess for signs of infection and treat promptly

  – **Teaching**

   * Explain prognosis and provide emotional support to family and child

  – **Emotional Care**

   * Promote normal growth and development for child

   * Discuss impact diagnosis has on child and family

f. **Potential Complications** — Infection, death.

10. WILM'S TUMOR (NEPHROBLASTOMA)

a. **Description** — A malignant, encapsulated tumor located in the kidney. It may also be accompanied by other congenital anomalies (genitourinary anomalies, aniridia). It usually affects the left kidney. It arises from embryonic tissue and is most often seen between 1 and 5 years, with peak incidence between 3 and 4 years of age. It is staged from 1-5 according to the growth and level of metastasis. It has a good prognosis especially for Stages 1-3.

b. **Signs and Symptoms** — Abdominal mass palpable (firm, nontender), increase in abdominal girth, hematuria, hypertension (25% of cases), anemia, pain and fever.

c. **Diagnostic Procedures** — Diagnosed by IV pyelogram, abdominal CT scan, presence of polycythemia, and urinalysis.

d. **Medical Interventions**

  – **Medications** — Administer chemotherapy according to specific protocols

  – **Treatments** — Administer radiation therapy

  – **Surgery** — Surgical removal of the kidney, adrenal gland and tumorous mass; other tissue which may be affected (lymph nodes) is also removed during this surgical procedure

e. **Nursing Interventions** — (See previous list of General Nursing Interventions)

  – **Assessment and Actions**

   * Avoid further palpation of the tumor before surgery

   * Provide postoperative care to child providing for comfort

- Teaching
  * Prepare family and child for surgery (usually within 24-48 hours after detection of tumor)
  * Prepare child and family for side effects of treatment regimen
  * Instruct family and child on importance of maintaining complete function of the remaining kidney, report signs of UTI or kidney infection promptly
- Emotional Care
  * Discuss impact diagnosis and treatment regimen have on family and child's life

f. **Potential Complications** — Infection, paralytic ileus (postoperatively), kidney failure or infection.

13

HEMATOLOGY DISORDERS

I. General Concepts

The major hematopoietic (blood forming) organs are red bone marrow and the lymphatic system
- **Plasma** — 90% water and 10% solutes (albumin, electrolytes, and proteins)
- **Cellular elements** — RBCs, WBCs, platelets

• Blood functions to bring oxygen to the tissues; buffer the fluid and electrolytes; repair injuries or infections, transport nutrients and waste products, and regulate the body's temperature

II. Specific Hematology Disorders

Congenital Disorders

1. COOLEY'S ANEMIA (BETA-THALASSEMIA MAJOR)

  a. **Description** — An autosomal co-dominant genetic trait in which there is diminished production of the beta globin chain of hemoglobin A causing severe anemia. It is primarily seen among the Black, Oriental and Mediterranean population. Typically the symptoms develop after six months of life. The child's bone marrow is hyperplastic and the RBCs are fragile. They seldom live until adulthood.

b. **Signs and Symptoms** — Severe anemia, hepatosplenomegaly jaundice, headache, anorexia, weakness, pallor, bone pain, flat bones of face characteristically widened, hemosiderosis, bronze skin appearance, fibrosis of major organs, (gallbladder, heart, liver, pancreas, spleen), delayed physical growth and sexual maturation.

c. **Diagnostic Procedures** — Diagnosed by CBC revealing anemia, hemoglobin electrophoresis shows elevated F and A hemoglobins.

d. **Medical Interventions**

   – **Medications** — Deferoxamine (iron-chelating agent given with Vitamin C; administer folic acid and testosterone; administer prophylactic antibiotic therapy postoperatively

   – **Treatments** — Blood transfusions as often as every three weeks

   – **Surgery** — Splenectomy may be necessary

e. **Nursing Interventions**

   – **Assessment and Actions**

      * Be alert to signs and symptoms indicating disorder

      * Assess child before, during and after transfusion (vital signs and signs of transfusion reactions)

      * Refer parents to genetic counseling

      * Observe for complications of multiple blood transfusions

   – **Teaching**

      * Explain diagnosis to parents and child and discuss treatment regimen

      * Discuss with parents the need for frequent transfusions

   – **Emotional Care**

      * Provide support to family and child in adjusting to a chronic illness

      * Support and facilitate grieving process

f. **Potential Complications** — Heart failure, diabetes, cirrhosis of the liver, cholelithiasis, hemosiderosis, death.

2. **HEMOPHILIA A (FACTOR VIII DEFICIENCY)**

   a. **Description** — A bleeding disorder, typically occurring in males, that is due to a deficiency in one of the normal clotting factors. The most common type (75%) is Hemophilia A in which Factor VIII is deficient. The severity of the disease ranges from mild to severe bleeding tendencies.

   b. **Signs and Symptoms** — Depend upon severity; frequent bruising or bleeding which is difficult to stop; hemarthrosis, epistaxis, internal and/or spontaneous hemorrhaging, joint pain and stiffness, hematuria.

   c. **Diagnostic Procedures** — Diagnosed by presence of abnormalities in blood clotting tests (PT, PTT, TGT, fibrinogen level) and absence or deficiency in Factor VIII assay.

d. **Medical Interventions**

- **Medications** — Corticosteroids are used judiciously to reduce inflammation of hemarthrosis

- **Treatments** — Administer (IV) missing Factor VIII; physical therapy to prevent loss of joint mobility; DDAVP, Ibuprofen

- **Surgery** — Unnecessary

e. **Nursing Interventions**

- **Assessment and Actions**

  * Be alert to signs and symptoms

  * Recognize and control bleeding

  * Obtain thorough history considering past bleeding episodes

  * Refer parents to genetic counseling

  * Monitor child's vital signs, and for reaction during transfusion

  * Assess for signs indicating potential complications

- **Teaching**

  * Explain diagnosis to parents and child and discuss treatment regimen

  * Explain administration of Factor VIII including frequency, duration and side effects

  * Explain how to prevent and control bleeding such as discouraging contact sports, utilizing soft toothbrush, maintaining normal weight for age to prevent further joint abuse, applying pressure to any cuts for 10 to 15 minutes as well as applying ice to area, immobilizing joints when swollen, and providing physical therapy once swelling reduced to maintain joint ROM

  * Prepare family for home care (self-administration of Factor VIII)

  * Teach methods for reducing discomfort (positioning, analgesics, application of cold or warmth)

- **Emotional Care**

  * Determine how parents and child are coping

  * Encourage child to discuss how disorder affects his life

  * Provide support to the family and child

  * Provide support group information to family

f. **Potential Complications** — Joint limitations, internal hemorrhaging, transfusion reactions, shock and death.

3. **HYPERBILIRUBINEMIA IN THE NEWBORN (NEWBORN JAUNDICE)**

a. **Description** — An overabundance of bilirubin in the blood stream. It often occurs in neonates (icterus neonatorum) and may be due to the immaturity of the liver or be due to Rh incompatibility (erythroblastosis fetalis).

b. **Signs and Symptoms** — Jaundice, elevated total bilirubin levels greater than 12 mg/dl.

c. **Diagnostic Procedures** — Diagnosed by assessing direct and indirect bilirubin levels, maternal blood group and Rh typing, and presence of positive direct and indirect Coomb's test.

d. **Medical Interventions**
   - **Medications** — Administer RhoGAM to mothers who are Rh negative to prevent this problem with successive births
   - **Treatments** — Administer phototherapy, monitor bilirubin levels, and possibly administer exchange transfusions (prn)
   - **Surgery** — Unnecessary

e. **Nursing Interventions**
   - **Assessment and Actions**
     * Assess newborn for jaundice by inspecting sclera and skin
     * If phototherapy used: cover infant's eyes and genitals in male; remove eye shields every feeding and when not under the lights; turn nude infant every 2 hours to expose all surface areas to light; maintain infant's temperature
     * Maintain hydration status of infant during therapy (frequent feedings and/or IV therapy)
     * Monitor bilirubin levels as ordered
     * If exchange transfusion utilized, monitor infant's vital signs, amount of blood removed and transfused, and for signs of reaction
     * Assess for signs of CNS changes (kernicterus) until level within normal range
   - **Teaching**
     * Explain diagnosis to parents and discuss treatment regimen
     * If home therapy utilized, instruct parents in care
   - **Emotional Care**
     * Encourage parents to care for and interact with child
     * Provide support and allow parents to ask questions

f. **Potential Complications** — Kernicterus/brain damage.

4. **SICKLE CELL ANEMIA**
   a. **Description** — An autosomal disorder in which hemoglobin A is replaced partly or completely by abnormal hemoglobin S which becomes sickled in shape when decreased oxygen is present. The sickled erythrocyte either hemolyzes or causes sluggish blood flow, thus decreasing its ability to carry oxygen. This disorder is usually found in the Black population but may also be present in individuals from the Arabian Peninsula, Greece, Turkey and India. Sickle cell anemia may be life threatening if a severe crisis occurs. Sickle cell trait is defined as those individuals who have less than 50% of HbS. People with sickle cell trait are typically asymptomatic unless under external stressors (vigorous exercise, illness, exposure to high altitudes) where oxygenation is diminished.

b. **Signs and Symptoms** — (Sickle Cell Crisis) mild to severe bone pain, acute abdominal arthralgia pain, low grade fever, hand-foot syndrome (pain and swelling in hands and feet); decreased growth; enlargement of spleen and liver; osteoporosis; priapism; ischemia may cause CVA and kidney malfunction.

c. **Diagnostic Procedures** — Diagnosed by presence of sickled RBC on blood smears, positive Sickledex, and evidence of sickling with hemoglobin electrophoresis.

d. **Medical Interventions**
   - **Medications** — Administer antibiotic for infection (if present), analgesics (PCA — Patient Controlled Analgesia) during sickle cell crisis
   - **Treatments** — Provide for adequate oxygenation, rest, hydration, and pain control measures; blood transfusions may be necessary
   - **Surgery** — Splenectomy may be necessary

e. **Nursing Interventions**
   - **Assessment and Actions**
     * Be alert to signs and symptoms
     * Refer parents to genetic counseling
     * During crisis promote oxygenation, hydration, bedrest
     * Provide method for reducing discomfort (warm compresses to area, elevating extremity)
   - **Teaching**
     * Explain diagnosis to parents and child and discuss treatment regimen
     * Teach parents and child how to prevent sickle cell crisis, treat infections promptly, maintain hydration status, avoid exercise that causes rapid oxygen depletion, diminish stressors
   - **Emotional Care**
     * Discuss chronicity of disease and how family is coping
     * Provide support to family and child
     * Provide information regarding support group

f. **Potential Complications** — CVA, blindness, cirrhosis of the liver, chronic ulceration of lower extremities, hepatomegaly, splenomegaly, heart failure, death.

Acquired Disorders

1. **IDIOPATHIC THROMBOCYTOPENIC PURPURA (ITP)**

   a. **Description** — An acute or chronic condition in which there is excessive damage and destruction of the platelets in the spleen. It is an autoimmune disorder. The acute form often follows an upper respiratory infection or communicable disease (rubella, varicella, or rubeola). Most children recover spontaneously.

b. **Signs and Symptoms** — Ecchymosis with petechiae, hematuria, hematemesis, bleeding gums, ecchymosis on lower extremities, epistaxis.

c. **Diagnostic Procedures** — Diagnosed by platelet count being <20,000/mm^3/dL; tourniquet test reveals petechiae formation.

d. **Medical Interventions**
   - **Medications** — Administer corticosteroids, gamma globulin
   - **Treatments** — Provide supportive care and safety since disorder is self-limiting; may require platelet transfusion if hemorrhaging occurs
   - **Surgery** — Usually unnecessary; splenectomy may be required for children with chronic disease

e. **Nursing Interventions**
   *See previous interventions for Hemophilia

   - **Assessment and Actions**
     * Be alert to signs and symptoms indicating disorder
     * Obtain thorough history to determine cause
     * Monitor for signs and symptoms of transfusion reaction
   - **Teaching**
     * Explain diagnosis to parents and discuss treatment regimen
     * Teach ways to prevent further bleeding episodes: omit contact sports or physical activity, maintain weight within normal limits, limit heavy lifting and stress to joints, utilize soft toothbrush, reduce chance for infection
     * Explain need for transfusion (prn)
   - **Emotional Care**
     * Provide parents and child time to ask questions and voice concerns
     * Provide support to family and child

f. **Potential Complications** — Transfusion reaction, hemorrhaging, shock, death if severe.

2. **IRON-DEFICIENCY ANEMIA**

   a. **Description** — A type of anemia which may be due to inadequate intake of iron (most common), increased iron needs, diminished iron stores, blood loss, or malabsorption. It is most commonly seen in infancy due to an over-consumption of milk and an iron-poor diet. It is most frequently seen in infants from 6 months to 3 years of age.

   b. **Signs and Symptoms** — Usually exhibits a gradual onset of signs and symptoms, underweight, overweight (milk baby), edema, limited activity level, retarded growth, fatigue, porcelain-like skin, paleness, muscle weakness, tachycardia, petechiae.

c. **Diagnostic Procedures** — Diagnosed by CBC which reveals hypochromic microcytic RBC, decreased hemoglobin, elevated RBC, decreased reticulocyte count, decreased serum iron concentration, and elevated total iron-binding capacity.

d. **Medical Interventions**

- **Medications** — Administer oral ferrous sulfate or IV iron dextran, administer ascorbic acid with iron to enhance GI absorption

- **Treatments** — Increase iron in diet, correcting underlying causes, and administer blood transfusion if severe anemia present

- **Surgery** — Unnecessary

e. **Nursing Interventions**

- **Assessment and Actions**

   * Be alert to signs and symptoms

   * Obtain thorough history to determine cause

   * Encourage rest periods and slowly increase activity level once child has begun treatment

   * Make parents aware that periodic screening may be done to assess child's progress

   * Assess for signs indicating potential complications

- **Teaching**

   * Prevent occurrence by encouraging iron supplements in infancy and including dark green leafy vegetables, red meats, organ meats or whole grains in child's diet

   * Explain diagnosis to family and discuss treatment regimen

   * Teach parents proper method of administering iron supplements: administer at back of mouth to prevent tooth staining, brush teeth after administration, administer with orange juice to enhance absorption

   * Warn parents stools may become darker with oral iron administration and child may become constipated; prevent constipation by exercising, high fiber diet, and increasing fluids

   * Instruct parents to decrease child's milk intake and provide other foods

- **Emotional Care**

   * Provide support to family and child

f. **Potential Complications** — Growth failure or delay, heart failure.

14

IMMUNE DISORDERS

I. General Concepts

- The immune system is composed of primary organs and secondary organs. Primary organs consist of the thymus (contains stem cells and T-lymphocytes) and marrow of long bones (contains stem cells for B-lymphocytes); secondary organs consist of the tonsils and adenoids, the lymph nodes which store both types of lymphocytes and filter antigens, and the spleen which filters antigens and initiates immune responses

- The immune system functions to protect the body against disease by: defending it against bacteria, viruses, parasites, toxins and other pathogenic agents; observing for and controlling rapid multiplication of abnormal cells (cancer); and clearing the body of the by-products of its own immune responses

- Intact skin and mucous membranes are the body's first line of defense. Also, acid gastric secretions, respiratory cilia, and the flushing action of urine help the body repel or destroy antigens

- The immune system provides nonspecific and specific immunity:

  - *Nonspecific immune response includes the body's ability to react to any foreign body regardless of previous exposure and is the first line of defense against an antigen.* The antigen produces an inflammatory response which in turn may produce fever, pain and purulence at the site: the process of phagocytosis and inflammation. An example of a nonspecific immune response would include the prodromal symptoms of communicable diseases

- *Specific immune responses are the body's final line of defenses in which the body responds to a specific antigen.* The immune response destroys the antigen and develops a memory that reactivates if the antigen appears again. This response is composed of cell mediated and humoral defense mechanisms. Each is specific against a unique antigen

  1. Cell-mediated response: T-lymphocyte mediated response
  2. Humoral mediated response: complement, B-lymphocytes and plasma cells (IgA, IgD, IgE, IgM, IgG) mediated response

- Immunity may be actively or passively-acquired and be a natural or artificial immunity (details in the Communicable Disease section)

- Immunological disorders may be due to a defect of the stem cell, T-cell, B-cell, or phagocyte

- The immune system may be affected by alterations in genetic make-up, nutrition, metabolism, anatomy or environmental factors

II. Specific Immune Disorders

Congenital Disorders

1. HUMORAL DEFICIENCIES

a. **Description** — Includes 3 major types of B cell alterations: congenital agammaglobulinemia, common variable deficiencies and selective immunoglobulin deficiencies.

Congenital agammaglobulinemia is an X-linked genetic disease that affects boys, produces a significant decrease in immunoglobulin levels or absence of several types of immunoglobulins and appears to prevent the development of B cells from stem cells.

Common variable deficiencies affect both genders equally and are deficiencies of more than one type of immunoglobulins due to nondifferentiation of B cells into immunoglobulin-producing plasma cells.

Selective immunoglobulin deficiencies usually affect only one class of immunoglobulins, usually IgA and IgM, and are seen in conjunction with autoimmune diseases.

The prognosis for children treated for humoral deficiencies is good, some children with IgA deficiency experience spontaneous resolution of the deficiency.

b. **Signs and Symptoms** — High susceptibility to bacterial infections, chronic respiratory infections, diarrhea. Some maternal antibody protection prevents major problems before early childhood but symptoms frequently appear when the child is very young. Children with common variable deficiency usually do not exhibit symptoms until later childhood.

  c. **Diagnostic Procedures** — Diagnosed by considering history of frequent and recurrent infections and assessing blood for low or nearly absent levels of IgG, IgA, or IgM, or all three. Levels of T-lymphocytes are usually normal. Plasma cells may be deficient except in X-linked agammaglobulinemia.

  d. **Medical Interventions**

    – **Medications** — Administer monthly intravenous immune globulin (IVIG) to children with congenital agammaglobulinemia and common variable deficiencies, 100-200 mg/kg. Immune globulin is not given to children with selective IgA deficiency because of the potential for precipitating an anti-IgA autoimmune reaction. Antibiotics are prescribed to treat infections and may be given prophylactically

    – **Treatments** — Provide child with clean environment, prevent and treat infections

    – **Surgery** — None recommended

  e. **Nursing Interventions**

    – **Assessment and Actions**

      * Administer IVIG slowly (see Potential Complications)

      * Obtain information about the number and types of infections the child has had

      * Assess the infection-prevention methods the family has used at home and what treatments have been successful

      * Help provide the child with a clean environment

      * Assess child's respiratory status

      * Assess for signs indicating potential complications

    – **Teaching**

      * Assess parents' and child's understanding of disease

      * Discuss ways to minimize infections (handwashing, maintaining thorough hygiene, prevent exposing child to others who are ill)

    – **Emotional Care**

      * Promote normal growth and development for age (see unit on Growth and Development)

      * Encourage child to discuss feelings

      * Determine family's level of coping and offer suggestions on ways to cope with situation

      * Provide support to family and child

  f. **Potential Complications** — Observe for signs/symptoms of an allergic reaction (urticaria), flushing, wheezing, dyspnea, or drop in blood pressure during IVIG administration. If any of these symptoms occur, stop the infusion, keep the line open and notify physician immediately. Keep epinephrine available during IVIG administration.

2. CELLULAR DEFICIENCY — DIGEORGE SYNDROME

a. **Description** — A rare disease of unknown origin that occurs during embryonic development. Primary defects are hypoplastic thymus and parathyroids, and defects in structures that are developing concurrently. These infants characteristically present with a small receding mandible, low-set ears, shortened upper lip and sometimes cleft lip and palate. Congenital cardiac anomalies may present with this diagnosis. Below normal or absent production of T-lymphocytes with this diagnosis affect the child's ability to fight infection but maternal antibody protection may delay appearance of infections. Prognosis is poor with a complete deficiency of T-lymphocytes.

b. **Signs and Symptoms** — Neonatal hypocalcemia and tetany are usually the first signs.

c. **Diagnostic Procedures** — Serum electrolytes to check for hypocalcemia and elevated phosphorus. Immunoglobulin levels are usually normal.

d. **Medical Interventions**
   - **Medications** — Intravenous calcium gluconate along with vitamin D
   - **Treatment** — Scrupulous handwashing and use of clean equipment, especially for feeding
   - **Surgery** — Thymic tissue transplants to establish cell-mediated immunity. Surgery may be required for cardiac anomalies

e. **Nursing Interventions**
   - **Assessment and Actions**
     * Initiate seizure precautions for the child with tetany
     * Monitor neurologic and cardiac status and prevent injury during seizures
     * Administer intravenous calcium carefully, observe for cardiac dysrhythmia and report to physician immediately
     * Prevent exposure to anyone with viral syndromes
     * Assess for signs indicating potential complications
   - **Teaching**
     * Assess parents' understanding of the disease
     * Discuss ways to minimize or avoid infections (handwashing and use of clean equipment, maintaining thorough hygiene, prevent exposing child to others who are ill)
   - **Emotional Care**
     * Promote normal growth and development for age (see unit on Growth and Development)
     * Counseling as needed for parental anxiety about child's prognosis
     * Financial counseling, if needed, since repeated hospitalizations are likely
     * Provide support to family and child

f. **Potential Complications** — Tetany can cause neurologic deficits with subsequent mental retardation. High concentrations of serum calcium during calcium administration may prevent relaxation of the heart muscle with subsequent hypertension, bradycardia and dysrhythmias.

3. **SEVERE COMBINED IMMUNODEFICIENCY SYNDROME (SCID)**

a. **Description** — A rare inherited disorder in which cellular and humoral immunity are absent or severely diminished. The prognosis is poor.

b. **Signs and Symptoms** — Extreme susceptibility to infections, especially opportunistic infections, vomiting, cough, *Candida* diaper rash, recurrence of infection or infections without complete recovery, FTT, diarrhea, thrush. With repeated severe infections, muscle wasting with diarrhea is a classic sign.

c. **Diagnostic Procedures** — Diagnoses by considering history of frequent and recurrent infections, and assessing blood for lymphocytopenia, presence of decreased plasma cells in bone marrow, and body's inability to respond to antigens.

d. **Medical Interventions**
   - **Medications** — Administer immunoglobulin, antibiotics given prophylactically to prevent *Pneumocystis* pneumonia
   - **Treatments** — Keep child in laminar airflow room or a plastic "bubble"
   - **Surgery** — Bone marrow transplantation has been successful in initiating both humoral and cellular immune response

e. **Nursing Interventions**
   - **Assessment and Actions**
     * Be alert for signs and symptoms indicating disorder
     * Provide child with sterile environment
     * Prevent and treat infections promptly
     * Refer parents to genetic counseling
     * If bone marrow transplant attempted, provide sterile environment and monitor child for signs of graft vs. host reaction (febrile episodes, diarrhea, hepatosplenomegaly, skin eruptions)
     * Assess for signs indicating potential complications
   - **Teaching**
     * Assess parents' and child's understanding of disease
     * Discuss ways to minimize infections (handwashing, maintaining thorough hygiene, prevent exposing child to others who are ill)
   - **Emotional Care**
     * Promote normal growth and development for age (see unit on Growth and Development)
     * Encourage child to discuss feelings

> * Determine family's level of coping and offer suggestions on ways to cope with situation
>
> * Provide support to family and child

f. Potential Complications — Graft vs. host reaction, which is irreversible, death from infections or transplant rejection.

Acquired Disorders

1. HUMAN IMMUNODEFICIENCY VIRUS (HIV) or ACQUIRED IMMUNODEFICIENCY SYNDROME (AIDS)

a. Description — This disorder is commonly referred to as AIDS, HIV, or HTLV 3. It is a chronic and often fatal disorder in which the body becomes infected by the Human T-cell Lymphotrophic virus. It is characterized by profound immunosuppression and results in susceptibility to opportunistic infection and neoplasms. HIV is transferred through blood and body fluids and is detectable in blood, semen, vaginal and cervical secretions, amniotic fluid, breast milk, alveolar fluid, saliva, tears, throat swabs and cerebrospinal fluid. Replication of the virus depends on viral and host factors. The progression of the disease in children is different from that of adults with children having a shorter latency period, 80% are symptomatic by age 2 years. The immature immune systems of infants may make them particularly susceptible to HIV.

b. Signs and Symptoms — FTT, frequent and recurrent oral monilial infections, generalized lymphadenopathy, hepatosplenomegaly, neurodevelopmental deficits, recurrent otitis media, parotid enlargement, rash.

c. Diagnostic Procedures — The principal manner of transmission in children is from mother to baby, so testing HIV-exposed infants is critical. The benefits of early identification include possible antiretroviral treatment, treatment for prevention of opportunistic infection, early intervention for problems related to growth and development and intervention for psychosocial-related problems. The principal manner of transmission in adolescents is blood, blood products and sexual contact. Children at risk are tested using the HIV antibody test. This test is not recommended for children under 18 months of age because of the presence of passively transferred maternal antibody in utero. For early detection of HIV in infants, the human immunodeficiency virus polymerase chain reaction (PCR) or HIV culture is most effective.

d. Medical Interventions

– **Medications** — Administer antiretroviral drugs, gamma globulin, antibiotics for infections

– **Treatments** — Directed toward decreasing the viral burden and alleviating opportunistic infections; augmenting the nutritional status, growth, development and general health; and treating chronic lung disease

– **Surgery** — Unnecessary

  e. **Nursing Interventions**

    – **Assessment and Actions** (similar to the assessment of a child with any immune deficiency)

      * Be alert to signs and symptoms of disorder

      * Determine mode of transmission and if others in family are HIV positive

      * Utilize Universal Precautions and encourage thorough hand-washing when in contact with child

      * Encourage well-balanced nutritional intake

      * Prevent child from being exposed to possible infections

      * Refer parents and child for counseling

    – **Teaching**

      * Explain diagnosis to parents and child (if appropriate for age) and how the disease is spread; explain it is *not* spread by hugging or kissing people; using the same toilet, tub, shower; sharing eating utensils; coughing or sneezing

      * Teach parents, care givers and child about nutrition and its role in maintaining health; encourage a well-balanced diet

      * Teach parents about medication prescribed (drug, dose, route, side effects)

      * Teach Universal Precautions to family members and care givers; avoid direct contact with blood, do not share personal items (like razors, toothbrushes, pierced earrings), open sores should be covered, use latex gloves when caring for child with bleeding, wash hands frequently when taking care of other bodily secretions

    – **Emotional Care**

      * Encourage expression of feelings

      * If mother was unaware of being HIV positive before her child was diagnosed, provide support and counseling for her

      * Promote child's development and growth

      * Enhance self-esteem and quality of child's life

      * Attempt to maintain routines in child's life

      * Promote positive family communication

      * Provide support to family and child, especially if extended family and other supports withdraw from contact with the family

      * Provide support group information to family

      * Help the family educate their community about HIV

  f. **Potential Complications** — Pneumonia, other opportunistic infections, skin lesions, often social isolation, and death.

2. **ANAPHYLAXIS**

  a. **Description** — A systemic allergic reaction to an extreme release of histamine and other chemical mediators. It can occur suddenly in response to an allergen that has not formerly elicited a reaction. Anaphylactic reactions usually occur as a result of an insect sting, administration of certain medications (especially antibiotics such as penicillin), allergy desensitization injections, or eating an allergenic food.

b. **Signs and Symptoms** — Initial symptoms include sneezing, generalized urticaria, weakness, restlessness, and severe anxiety. These are followed by laryngeal spasms and edema, gastrointestinal symptoms, dyspnea, severe hypotension, increased pulse, and pallor or cyanosis. If untreated, death occurs from an occluded airway and vascular collapse. Anaphylactic reactions can occur from seconds to almost 30 minutes after exposure to an allergen.

c. **Diagnostic Procedures** — Diagnosed by rapid onset of symptoms, physical findings and history.

d. **Medical Interventions**
   - **Medications** — Depend upon severity but may include administration of diphenhydramine (mild reaction), epinephrine or aminophylline administration
   - **Treatments** — Provide supportive care (oxygen, airway maintenance, IV fluids) for a patient in shock; ventilation may be necessary
   - **Surgery** — Unnecessary

e. **Nursing Interventions**
   - Assessment and Actions
     * Be alert to signs and symptoms as prompt detection may be life-saving for child
     * Monitor vital signs, respiratory status, neurological status, and I&O
     * Assist with administration of medication as ordered
     * Identify allergen to which exposed and instruct parents and child to attempt to prevent further exposure, if possible
     * Encourage child to wear a MedicAlert bracelet or tag
     * Alert teachers, school nurse, and friends of possible allergen, signs of reactions and treatment regimen
   - **Teaching**
     * Explain diagnosis to parents and child and discuss treatment regimen
     * Teach parents how to recognize future reactions and treat by carrying and using diphenhydramine or epinephrine injector
   - **Emotional Care**
     * Provide support to family and child

f. **Potential Complications** — Coma or death if untreated.

APPENDIX A
Growth Charts

Girls: Birth to 36 months
Physical Growth NCHS Percentiles*

Girls: Birth to 36 months
Physical Growth NCHS Percentiles*

DATE	AGE	LENGTH	WEIGHT	HEAD CIRC.	COMMENT

SIMILAC® WITH IRON
Infant Formula

ISOMIL®
Soy Protein Formula with Iron

Reprinted with permission
of Ross Laboratories

Girls: Prepubescent
Physical Growth NCHS Percentiles*

Adapted from: Hamill PVV, Drizd TA, Johnson CL, Reed RB, Roche AF, Moore WM. Physical growth: National Center for Health Statistics percentiles. AM J CLIN NUTR 32:607-629, 1979. Data from the National Center for Health Statistics (NCHS) Hyattsville, Maryland

© 1982 Ross Laboratories

SIMILAC® WITH IRON
Infant Formula

ISOMIL®
Soy Protein Formula with Iron

Reprinted with permission
of Ross Laboratories

Girls: 2 to 18 years
Physical Growth NCHS Percentiles*

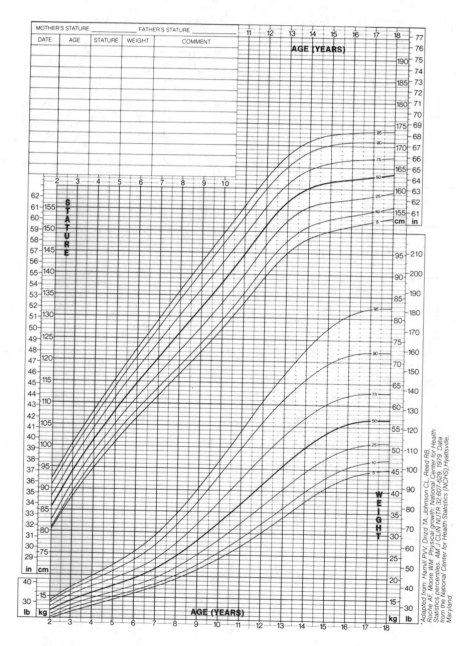

Boys: Birth to 36 months
Physical Growth NCHS Percentiles*

Boys: Birth to 36 months
Physical Growth NCHS Percentiles*

DATE	AGE	LENGTH	WEIGHT	HEAD CIRC.	COMMENT

SIMILAC® WITH IRON
Infant Formula

ISOMIL®
Soy Protein Formula with Iron

*Adapted from: Hamill PVV, Drizd TA, Johnson CL, Reed RB, Roche AF, Moore WM: Physical growth: National Center for Health Statistics percentiles. AM J CLIN NUTR 32:607-629, 1979. Data from the Fels Longitudinal Study, Wright State University School of Medicine, Yellow Springs, Ohio.

© 1982 Ross Laboratories

Reprinted with permission of Ross Laboratories

Boys: Prepubescent
Physical Growth NCHS Percentiles*

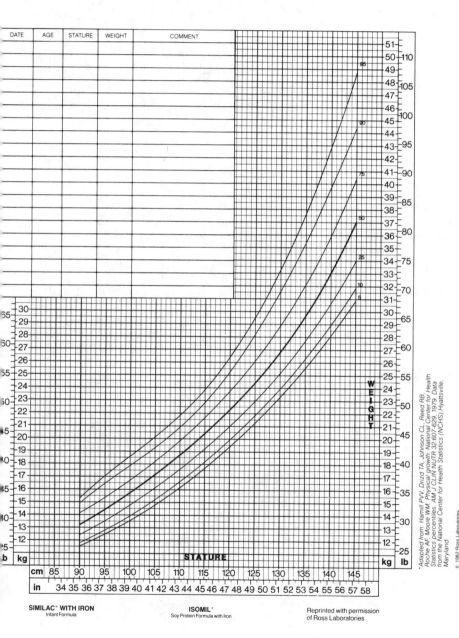

Boys: 2 to 18 years
Physical Growth NCHS Percentiles*

Ross
Growth &
Development
Program

APPENDIX B
Growth and Development Assessment

This growth and development chart is an assessment of major developmental milestones at a specific age. This is essential information for anyone who assesses children.

BIRTH - 4 MONTHS
* Startle response to noise
* Turns head to direction of voice
* Smiles at another
* Cries to express displeasure (2 weeks)
* Stops crying when parent enters the room (1-3 months)
* Grasps at objects when placed in hand
* Holds head up momentarily (4 weeks)
* Begins to hold head constantly (16 weeks)
* Will follow toy within line of sight
* Laughs out loud (16 weeks)
* Stares at own hands
* Looks at himself in mirror
* Vocalizes when talked to (12 weeks)

4 - 6 MONTHS
* Recognizes familiar sounds, recognizes voices
* Reaches for objects, but often misjudges distance
* Full control of head movements
* Enjoys playing with toys
* Sits if propped
* Sits in highchair (6 months)
* Rolls from prone to supine
* Pulls up to sit
* Plays peek-a-boo
* Begins to differentiate likes and dislikes of food
* Imitates several sounds (4 months)
* Spontaneous vocal-social behavior (6 months)

6 - 9 MONTHS
* Drinks from cup
* Eats solid foods
* Responds to name
* Responds to gestures (bye-bye, pat-a-cake)
* Puts things in mouth
* Says "da" and "bye"

* Feeds self cookie
* Transfers objects hand-to-hand
* May imitate adults
* Rolls from supine to prone
* Becomes fretful when mother leaves, apprehensive of strangers
* Responds to own name (9 months)
* Able to show emotions: anger, frustration, affection, fear, anxiety, pleasure

9 - 12 MONTHS

* Imitates voice sounds
* Speaks first real words
* Offers head and foot while dressing
* Creeps
* Comprehends meaning of mama, dada, bye, no
* Rolls ball to another person
* Shows pincer grasp
* Pulling to standing position

12 - 15 MONTHS

* Enjoys rhymes
* Identifies objects
* Responds to simple commands
* Begins to recognize wet diaper
* Kisses upon request
* Begins to develop a memory
* May exhibit shyness
* Jabbers in non-meaningful sentences
* Walks with assistance (13 months)
* Drinks from cup, feeds self
* Takes off shoes
* Points at things he wants
* Babinski's reflex

15 - 18 MONTHS

* Walks without assistance
* Understands simple instructions
* Uses "no" indiscriminately
* Gains sphincter control
* Temper tantrums more evident
* Kisses and hugs
* Anterior fontanel closes by 18 months

18 - 24 MONTHS

* Listens to simple stories

* Vocabulary increases to 300 words
* Produces word combinations
* Refers to himself by name
* Runs and falls
* Throws ball without falling
* Begins to scribble
* Points to nose, hair
* Asks for food, drinks
* Washes hands
* Builds tower of blocks
* Turns pages of book
* Puts on clothes, shoes
* Talks constantly
* Parallel play (watches others play but does not play with them)
* Height at 24 months approximately 1/2 of adult

24 - 30 MONTHS

* Talks in phases
* Turns doorknob
* Takes off lids
* Begins to draw
* Knows first and last name
* Talks constantly
* Has imaginary playmate
* Attention span increasing
* Dresses self
* Listens to 5-10 minute story (30 months)

3 YEARS

* Rapid expansion of vocabulary (900 words)
* Identifies objects and what they are for
* Carries on conversation
* Uses simple sentences
* Night-time bladder control
* Learns to ride tricycle
* Uses scissors, copies a square
* Asks questions constantly
* Expresses fear of dark
* Realizes own sex
* Parallel and associative play

4 YEARS

* Girls are a little ahead of boys in language development

* Vocabulary extends to 1500 words
* Receptive vocabulary comparable to expressive vocabulary of adult
* Fewer grammatical errors
* Exaggerates stories
* Constantly questioning
* Becoming independent
* Strongly attached to parent of opposite sex
* Associative and cooperative play

5 YEARS

* Vocabulary of 2,000 words
* Can count up to ten
* Knows his age
* Knows primary colors
* Sentences more complex
* Aware of handedness
* Ties shoelaces
* Names money
* Can follow 3 instructions at a time
* Eager to please
* Identifies with parent of same sex
* Cooperative play
* Height and weight gain slower
* More trustworthy and responsible

6 YEARS

* Sentences grammatically correct
* Reads simple stories
* Tends to giggle over nothing
* Aware of days and seasons
* Gaining more independence
* Imitates adults more
* Knows left from right, AM from PM

APPENDIX C
Health Assessment Tips

Environment
* Quiet, private area
* Temperature of comfort for client
* No bright lights or glare from sun
* Provide comfort, security for client: infants and toddlers — on mother's lap; preschooler, schoolage — mother at side; adolescent — determine whether prefers parents' presence; provide confidentiality, privacy and reassure

Introduction
* Address child and parent; use child's name frequently
* Explain reason for interview, what will happen
* Establish rapport with child using gentle touch, eye contact, speaking to child at eye level
* Assure that information will be kept confidential
* Postpone interview if client is in pain or agitated
* Be attentive and avoid interruptions

Age-related Techniques
* Obtain most of information from parent or reliable source (child's memory is often inaccurate)
* Repeat statements and questions if necessary, allow time to respond
* Incorporate children over 2 years in simple questions to give a sense of control
* Allow for frequent questions; explain in simple terms

Communication Techniques
* Develop rapport — give individual attention, look at child and family, listen, give encouragement
* Be aware of verbal and nonverbal cues (yours and child's parents')
* Use open-ended and direct questions; avoid leading questions
* Clarify as needed

APPENDIX D
Health Assessment

Reason for Contact
Biographical Data
- Patient's name, address, telephone number
- Age
- Date of birth
- Sex
- Primary language spoken
- Names of parents, care providers
- Source of data (informant) and reliability

Present Illness History
(if child presents with an illness or concern, either physical, psychological or social)
- Onset, location, quality and quantity of discomfort, aggravating and alleviating factors, how has complaint impacted child's life/activity level; treatments (including medications) and response to treatment; reason for seeking health care

Past History
- Birth
  * Prenatal — Mother's general state of health while pregnant; complications during pregnancy (medications taken, illnesses, accidents); was this a planned pregnancy; number of pregnancies, births, abortions, miscarriages
  * Natal — Length of pregnancy (gestational age), where delivered, difficulty with labor, type of delivery, condition of baby at birth, birth weight, APGAR score, complications
  * Postnatal — Complications: jaundice, cyanosis, oxygen requirement, respirator, feeding problems, infections; how long in hospital
- Allergies
  * Medications, animals, foods, environmental, latex: identify type of reaction
- Accidents
  * Type, age occurred, treatment, sequelae, child's reaction
- Illnesses
  * Childhood diseases: measles, mumps, varicella, etc. and any complications, or sequelae
- Hospitalizations/Operations
  * Specify type, reason for, outcome, child's reaction, follow-up needed, any complications or sequelae

- Immunizations
  * Current immunization status for age, previous adverse reactions
- Current Medications
  * Name, dose, schedule, duration, reason for taking; include vitamins, over-the-counter medications, herbal preparations
- Habits
  * Diet — Typical day (24 hour), type, amount, supplements, weight gain/loss
  * Sleep — Number of hours, naps, sleep problems
  * Elimination — Bowel/bladder patterns, toilet trained, bedwetting
  * Growth and Development — Identify developmental milestones, age-appropriate (physical, social, cognitive, emotional); any difficulties; special concerns, learning problems, school performance; personality of child, usual habits (pacifier, thumbsucking); peer relationships; use of tobacco/drugs; screening exams: dental, vision, hearing, developmental
- Review of Systems
  * General — Weight loss/gain, chronic fevers
  * Head — Size, fontanels, masses, trauma, headaches
  * Skin — Pruritis, eczema, rashes, deformities of nails, hair, skin; bruising, petechiae, birthmarks, cyanosis, edema
  * Eyes — Vision problems, color vision, strabismus, cataract, corrective devices, infections
  * Ears — Hearing loss, otitis media, speech
  * Nose — Recurrent nosebleeds, sinus infections, ability to smell, drainage, patency, runny or stuffy nose, nasal discharge
  * Mouth and Throat — Infections, tonsillitis, strep throats, number and color of teeth, cavities, adenotonsillar hypertrophy, bifid uvula, difficulty swallowing, chewing, hoarseness
  * Neck — Pain, limitation of movement, masses, stiffness, thyroid enlargement, enlarged lymph nodes
  * Chest/Respiratory — Breast enlargement, masses, discharge, shape of chest; chronic cough dyspnea, wheezing, bronchitis/bronchiolitis, pneumonia, stridor, hemoptysis, number of colds per year, tuberculosis, perform self breast exam (adolescents)
  * Cardiovascular — Pallor, cyanosis, fainting episodes, hyper or hypotension, known cardiac defects, exercise intolerance, feeding difficulty, murmurs, anemia
  * Gastrointestinal — Appetite, constipation, nausea, vomiting, diarrhea, distention, problems with liver, jaundice, abdominal pain, change in habits, ulcers, gastroesophageal reflux (GER), colitis
  * Genitourinary — Frequency, dysuria, hematuria, polyuria, incontinence, discharge, infections, difficulty with stream, testes descended, testicular, scrotal or inguinal swelling, testicular self examination

* Gynecological — Menarche, date of last menstrual period (LMP), sexually-transmitted diseases, difficulty with menses, vaginal discharge, PAP smear, if sexually active type of contraception used, obstetric history, if appropriate

* Musculoskeletal — Strength/weakness, numbness, injuries, stiffness, limited ROM, congenital disorders, gait problems, fractures, arthritis, symmetry, paralysis, pain

* Neurological — Headaches, seizures, syncope, breathholding, coordination, loss of memory, unusual behaviors (aggressive, combative, withdrawn), change in level of consciousness, headaches, learning problems

* Chronic — Growth pattern, excessive thirst, diaphoresis, presence of sexual characteristics, chronic fevers, unusual bruising/bleeding

Family History

- Family Profile

  * Names and ages of each member of the family

  * Health status of each family member

  * Age of onset of illnesses in family

  * Family interaction

  * Family support systems

  * Cultural background

  * Utilization of the health care system

  * Health beliefs, practices

  * Family stresses

- Family Medical History

  * Review of systems for the child's maternal and paternal sides of the family; identify any potentially inherited disorders: diabetes, asthma, epilepsy, syndromes, glaucoma, cataracts, heart disease, mental retardation, mental illnesses, cystic fibrosis, hemophilia, von Willebrand's disease, cancer, muscular dystrophy, multiple sclerosis, lupus, etc.

APPENDIX E
Physical Assessment

Environment
- Provide well-lighted setting
- Decrease noise and distractions
- Ensure safety for infant, child/parent
- Provide for privacy
- Properly drape for privacy, utilize extra blanket for warmth
- Warm hands and instruments before touching client
- Place client in sitting or supine position depending on system being examined
- Allow to empty bladder before examination

Procedures for Examination
Infant and Toddler
- Introduce self
- Allow parent or caretaker to hold infant or child when possible
- Utilize a slow approach and establish rapport with child and parent
- Allow parent to assist with positioning when necessary to allow a sense of control
- Obtain "quiet" vital signs and assessment items that require auscultation first (respirations and lung fields, apical pulse, heart sounds, and abdominal sounds)
- Remember that obtaining blood pressure and temperature may cause discomfort. This may be done after need for silence is over
- Utilize play and interact with client to maintain rapport
- Perform exam on parent's lap if child prefers
- Examine eyes, ears, nose, throat last
- Talk with parent or caretaker in a soft, gentle voice throughout exam explaining each area being assessed
- Maintain normal temperature throughout exam by keeping infant/toddler in a blanket or sheet and assessing one area at a time
- Answer all questions and concerns, inform of use of information
- Inform if any further examination needed
- Discuss findings with parent
- Provide educational information to parent, prn
- Use toys to distract child while examining

Preschooler
- Introduce self, establish rapport
- Explain each portion of exam in simple terms before performing
- Place child in a position near parent that is safe
- Assess the child interacting at eye level

- Approach slowly, examine in a toe-to-head direction leaving eyes, ears, nose, throat for last
- Assess "quiet" vital signs and areas first (respirations and lung fields, apical pulse, heart sounds, and abdominal sounds) before invasive procedures are assessed
- Describe to child what blood pressure will feel like to reduce surprise effect
- Describe to child how they may assist with exam
- Have parent assist with undressing child; provide a drape for privacy
- Allow preschooler to examine equipment prior to use, to alleviate anxiety
- Perform exam on parent's lap if child prefers
- Stress normal findings throughout exam
- Apply a Band-Aid over invasive procedures which injure the skin
- Discuss findings with parent
- Provide educational information to parent, prn
- Answer all questions and concerns, inform if any further examination needed

School-Age
- Introduce self
- Establish rapport
- Explain procedures to child/parent
- Describe length of time exam will take and child's role
- Position child safely on exam table or bed with parent in room
- Ask if child has any questions before beginning exam, during exam, at completion of exam
- Assess all vital signs first
- Perform physical assessment in a head-to-toe sequence, save genitalia until last if child is shy or anxious
- Provide privacy, drape child as each area is assessed
- Stress normal findings
- Discuss results with child/parent
- Provide educational background
- Answer all questions and concerns, inform of use of information
- Inform if any further examination needed
- Invite to participate in care plan if interested

Adolescent
- Introduce self, establish rapport
- Determine whether client wants parent in exam room
- Explain each procedure and teenager's role in assisting with examination
- Encourage questions, comments or concerns to be mentioned throughout exam
- Provide for privacy
- Perform assessment in a head-to-toe process
- Stress normal findings

- Perform genital exam at end of assessment; talk/explain procedure in quiet voice as each area palpated and inspected
- Answer all questions and concerns, inform of use of information
- Inform if any further examination needed
- Invite to participate in care plan if interested
- Provide educational information to adolescent and parent, prn

APPENDIX F
Physical Assessment

Vital Signs
- Temperature
- Pulse
- Respiration
- Blood pressure

Measurements
- Height/length
- Weight
- Head and chest circumference (if age appropriate)

General Condition
- Appearance
- Behavior
- Activity
- Nutrition
- Hygiene

Skin
- Color
- Moisture
- Texture
- Temperature
- Turgor
- Hair
- Nails
- Lesions (color, distribution, shape, type, size)

Lymph nodes
- Palpable nodes
- Size
- Tenderness
- Shape
- Mobility
- Normal findings include: palpable nodes not greater than 3 mm except in cervical and groin area where may be 1 cm

Head
- Shape
- Masses
- Size
- Symmetry
- Fontanels
- Sutures

- Lesions
- Position of eyes, ears, nose and mouth
- Abnormalities

Eyes

- Shape
- Symmetry
- Lids
- Lashes
- Moisture
- Coordination (nystagmus or strabismus)
- Exudate
- PEARLA
- Visual acuity

Ears

- Placement
- Shape
- Drainage
- Masses
- Lesions
- Foreign bodies
- Tympanic membrane (pull ear down and back in children under the age of three — color, light reflex, bony landmarks, intact)

Nose

- Placement
- Patency
- Lesions
- Drainage
- Masses
- Respiratory effort
- Obstruction

Mouth

- Color
- Moisture
- Lesions
- Lips
- Placement and size of internal structures (tongue, uvula, palates, teeth)
- Number and appearance of teeth
- Color of mucosa
- Odor

Throat

- Color
- Tonsils
- Exudate

Neck
- Symmetry
- Masses
- ROM
- Webbing
- Pulsations
- Size of thyroid

Chest
- Shape
- Masses
- Bilateral symmetry
- Pulsations
- Respiratory effort and type (diaphragmatic or abdominal breathing), retractions
- Breast development and placement

Lungs
- Breath sounds (intensity, quality, duration)
- Sounds on inspiration and/or expiration (clear, crackles, rhonchi, wheezing, pleural rub)
- Bilaterally equal chest expansion

Heart
- Pulses equal in rate and intensity in all extremities
- Temperature and color of extremities
- Heart sounds (rate, rhythm, murmurs)
- PMI
- Clubbing
- Palpations
- Activity level
- Edema
- Cyanosis

Abdomen
- Size
- Shape
- Symmetry
- Masses
- Visible peristaltic activity
- Bowel sounds
- Appearance of umbilicus
- Abdominal girth
- Tenderness
- Rigidity
- Guarding
- Rebound tenderness

- Palpable liver
- Spleen
- Bladder
- Kidney

Genitalia
*Female:
- Presence and position of urethra, labia, vagina
- Exudate
- Lesions
- Masses
- Pubic development/Tanner's stage

*Male:
- Position and shape of penis
- Urethra
- Scrotum
- Testes
- Exudate
- Lesions
- Masses
- Pubic development/Tanner's stage

Rectum/Anus
- Patency
- Lesions
- Muscle tone
- Stools
- Masses

Musculoskeletal
- Gait
- Posture
- Stance
- Coordination
- Symmetry in muscle size and tone
- Strength
- Masses
- Spinal alignment
- Pilonidal dimples
- Long bone alignment
- Joints (ROM, tenderness, warmth, edema)
- Dislocations
- Hand/palm/foot appearance (palmar/plantar creases, webbing of fingers, number of fingers/toes)

Nervous system
- Alertness
- Activity level
- Coordination
- Motor development
- Cranial nerves
- Reflexes
- Cerebellar functions
- Sensory functions

APPENDIX G
Medication Tables

The following medication charts include the commonly prescribed medications for children. In addition to dosages specific to pediatrics, the author has placed special emphasis on nursing actions and patient teaching.

Table 1. ANALGESICS AND SEDATIVES

Name	Uses	Route and Dose	Adverse Reactions/ Side Effects	Drug or Food Interactions	Nursing Considerations
Generic: Acetaminophen **Trade:** Tylenol, Tempra,	Non-narcotic analgesic/antipyretic used for relief of mild to moderate pain and control of fever.	**Infants & Children:** Oral: 10-15 mg/kg/dose every 4-6 hrs as needed; may repeat doses 4-5 times/day; do not exceed 5 doses in 24 hrs. Rectal: 10-15 mg/kg/dose every 4-6 hrs as needed **Adults:** Oral, rectal: 325-650 mg every 4-6 hrs, not to exceed 4 g/day	**CNS:** Mental confusion, lethargy, seizures **Hepatic:** Liver damage with abnormal liver function tests with 2-4 days of overdose **GU:** Hematuria, renal damage and dysfunction (more common in children with renal disease) **Skin:** Rash, urticaria **Hemic:** Bleeding, echymosis, anemia, thrombocytopenia, leukopenia (more common with long-term use) **Other:** Anaphylaxis	**Drugs:** Alcohol and other heptatoxic drugs; decreased action with chronic barbiturate use; increased anticoagulant effect of coumarin with chronic use; increased nephrotoxicity if combined with long-term aspirin use; potential for hypothermia if used with phenothiazines. **Food:** Decreased absorption if taken with a high carbohydrate meal.	* Note hepatic and renal function and monitor if long-term use anticipated. * May be crushed and given with food. * Patient/parent education includes: - Do not give with any other OTC medication. - If illness lasts >3 days or no relief obtained, consult MD. - Limit to 5 doses/day.
Generic: Chloral Hydrate **Trade:** Aquachloral, Noctec	Hypnotic used preoperatively to reduce anxiety, postoperatively with analgesics, and for sedation prior to tests such as CT scan and MRI.	**Oral, rectal:** **Neonates:** 25 mg/kg/dose for sedation prior to a procedure **Children:** Sedation, anxiety: 15-50 mg/kg/dose every 4-6 hrs Hypnotic: 50 mg/kg/dose Nonpainful procedures requiring sedation: 50-100 mg/kg and repeat the dose to a max of 120 mg/kg total (max: 2 G total dose) if the child is not sleeping within 30 mins after the first dose; give first dose 30-60 mins before procedure **Adults:** Sedation, anxiety: 250 mg 3 times/day Hypnotic: 500-1000 mg at bedtime or 30 minutes prior to the procedure, not to exceed 2 G/24 hrs	**CNS:** Continued sedation, disorientation, paranoia, paradoxical excitement, headache **CV:** Dysrhythmias with overdose, bradycardia **Respiratory:** Depression with overdose **Hepatic:** Jaundice with overdose **Hemic:** Leukopenia, eosinophilia	**Drugs:** CNS depressants potentiate this medication; causes diaphoresis, flushing, and hypertension when given with IV furosemide; hypoprothrombinemia when given with oral anticoagulants, particularly warfarin **Food:** None	* Obtain baseline vital signs. * PO may be given with food to decrease gastric distress. * Check anal area prior to administering PR dose. * Put side rails up after administration and keep potentially dangerous items away from patient. * Observe for onset of sleep. * Monitor for signs of overdose (hypotension, weakness, coma, dysrhythmias, vomiting). * Patient/parent education: - Avoid driving and performing other potentially dangerous tasks while taking this medication. - Avoid taking with other medications unless directed by physician.

Name	Uses	Route and Dose	Adverse Reactions/ Side Effects	Drug or Food Interactions	Nursing Considerations

Generic: Codeine
 	
Trade: Combined with other products such as Tylenol, phenergan, and guiatussin
	Narcotic analgesic, opiate agonist, antitussive used to treat mild to moderate pain and suppress cough.	Analgesic: Oral:
		Children: 0.5-1 mg/kg/dose every 4-6 hrs as needed; maximum: 60 mg/dose.
		Adults: 15-60 mg every 4-6 hrs as needed.
		
		Antitussive: Oral:
		Children:
		2-6 yrs: 2.5-5 mg every 4-6 hrs as needed; maximum: 30 mg/day.
		7-12 yrs: 5-10 mg every 4-6 hrs as needed; maximum: 60 mg/day, or 1-1.5 mg/kg/day in divided doses every 4-6 hrs as needed.
		Adults: 10-20 mg/dose every 4-6 hrs as needed; maximum 120 mg/day.
			CNS: Sedation, restlessness, insomnia
			CV: Circulatory depression, orthostatic hypotension, palpitation, brady- or tachycardia
			GI: Nausea, vomiting, constipation
			Resp: Respiratory depression is a serious side effect
			Hepatic: Biliary spasm, increased serum amylase and lipase
			GU: Urinary retention, oliguria, impotence
			Skin: Rash, erythema, urticaria, pruritus, facial flushing
				Drug: Potentiated by CNS depressants such as alcohol; incompatible with aminophylline, heparin, methicillin, phenobarbital, sodium bicarbonate; decreases effects of diuretics in congestive heart failure.
				
				Food: None
					* Assess type and degree of pain prior to administration.
					* Use other pain control methods in addition to analgesics.
					* Take baseline vital signs.
					* Give PO forms with food to decrease gastric distress.
					* Rotate injection sites.
					* Raise side rails.
					* Monitor vital signs q 15-30 minutes following administration.
					* Evaluate amount of pain within 30 minutes following administration.
					* Patient/parent education:
					  - Take drug only as directed and only for patient prescribed .
					  - Drug may cause drowsiness; avoid driving and adjust other activities accordingly.
					  - Do not administer to child <1 yr or extended release forms to child < 6 yr.
					  - Observe for excessive drowsiness.

Name	Uses	Route and Dose	Adverse Reactions/ Side Effects	Drug or Food Interactions	Nursing Considerations

Generic: Diazepam
 	
Trade: Valium
	Sedative and anticonvulsant used as an anti-anxiety agent and to treat generalized seizures.	PO:
		Sedative or muscle relaxant: 0.12-0.8 mg/kg/day equally divided q 6-8 h
		
		IM, IV:
		Sedative or muscle relaxant: 0.04-0.2 mg/kg/dose q 2-4 h (max dose = 0.6 mg/kg within 8 h)
		
		Status Epilepticus:
		1 mo - 5 yrs: 0.2-0.5 mg/kg/dose IV every 2-5 mins up to a maximum of 5 mg
		>5 yrs: 1 mg every 2-5 mins until a max of 10 mg
		Rectal: 0.5 mg/kg, then 0.25 mg/kg in 10 mins if needed
		Adolescents: Conscious sedation for procedures: Oral: 10 mg; IV: 5 mg, may repeat with 2.5 mg
			CNS: Drowsiness, paradoxical excitement, dizziness, ataxia, confusion, weakness, tremor, vertigo, syncope
			CV: Hypotension, brady-cardia, cardiac arrest with rapid IV infusion
			GI: Nausea, vomiting, constipation, diarrhea, appetite and weight changes, increased salivation, metallic taste, decreased gag reflex
			Resp: Apnea with rapid IV infusion
			GU: Retention, incontinence
			Skin: Rash, urticaria, pruritus, photosensitivity
			Musculoskeletal: Bone pain, muscle cramps, paresthesia
			Sensory: Blurred vision, nystagmus, diplopia
				Drugs: Increased CNS depressant effects if given with other CNS depressants; lowered seizure threshold with tricyclic antidepressants; decreased clearance and increased levels if taken with cimetidine and disulfiram; increased hypotension with other drugs that have this effect; decreased absorption with antacids; reduced digoxin excretion; enhanced excretion with refampin; increased phenytoin levels; potentiate MAO inhibitors.
				
				Food: None
					* Take baseline vital signs.
					* May give po forms with a small amount of food.
					* Incompatible with other drugs; do not mix if giving IV.
					* Interacts with plastic - give as close to vein as is possible.
					* Avoid extravasation.
					* Monitor CBC, liver function tests, nutrition and weight if on long-term therapy.
					* Patient/parent education:
					  - Take drug only as directed and only for patient prescribed.
					  - Drug may cause drowsiness; avoid driving, adjust other activities accordingly.
					  - Avoid OTC drugs, alcohol, other illicit drugs.
					  - Report drowsiness, dizziness, excitement or other unusual effects to MD.
					  - Wear identification if taking this medication for seizure control.
					* Administer IV push over 3-5 mins; maximum concentration 5 mg/ml

Name	Uses	Route and Dose	Adverse Reactions/ Side Effects	Drug or Food Interactions	Nursing Considerations
Generic: Fentanyl Citrate Trade: Sublimaze	Acts as a general anesthetic in higher doses and as analgesic for moderate to severe pain in lower doses.	IV: 1-4 mcg/kg/dose slow IV push repeated q 2-4h prn. Infants: Analgesia: 1 mcg/kg/ dose; may repeat every 1-2 hrs Infusion: 2-5 mcg/kg/hour Children: Sedation for procedures/ analgesia: IM, IV: 1-3 yrs: 2-3 mcg/kg/ dose 3 mins before procedure; may repeat after 30-60 mins 3-12 yrs: 1-2 mcg/kg/ dose 3 mins before procedure; may repeat after 30-60 mins Continuous analgesia: 1-3 mcg/kg/hour Analgesia: IV: 0.5-2 mcg kg every 1-2 hrs	CNS: Dizziness, sedation, weakness, restlessness, insomnia, seizures CV: Bradycardia, hypotension GI: Nausea, vomiting, abdominal cramps, constipation Resp: Respiratory depression, atelectasis, dyspnea GU: Oliguria, urinary retention Skin: Itching, rash, hives	Drugs: Potentiated by other drugs having the same effect; increased hypotensive effect with antihypertensives; benzodiazepines may increase amount of fentanyl needed; excitement and hypertension if given within 14 days of MAO inhibitors. Food: None	* Obtain baseline vital signs and reassess frequently with particular attention paid to respiratory rate and effort. * Patient/parent education: - Cough and deep breathe frequently. - Stay in bed with side rails up. * Administer slow IV push over 3-5 minutes or by infusion. * Continuous pulse oximeter recommended during adminis-tration.

Name	Uses	Route and Dose	Adverse Reactions/ Side Effects	Drug or Food Interactions	Nursing Considerations
Generic: Ibuprofen **Trade:** Motrin, PediaProfen	Nonsteroidal anti-inflammatory, analgesic, antipyretic used for mild to moderate pain, control of fever, and to treat rheumatoid arthritis.	Infants and children: Antipyretic: 10 mg/kg/dose divided every 6-8 hrs for fever >102°F or fever resistant to acetaminophen Juvenile Rheumatoid Arthritis: 30-70 mg/kg/day or 850-2100 mg/m2/24 hrs; usual dose is 50 mg/kg/24 hrs or 1600 mg/m2/24 hrs divided every 6 hrs Analgesic: 4-10 mg/kg/ dose every 6-8 hrs	**CNS:** Dizziness, headache, confusion, depression **CV:** Fluid retention, CHF, hypertension, palpation, dysrhythmias **GI:** Nausea, vomiting, heartburn **Resp:** Bronchospasm, dyspnea **Hepatic:** Jaundice, hepatitis, altered liver enzymes **GU:** Polyuria, hematuria, renal failure **Hemic:** Inhibited platelet action, prolonged bleeding time, neutropenia, thrombocytopenia, anemia **Sensory:** Blurred or disturbed vision, tinnitus	**Drugs:** Increased renal side effects with acetaminophen and diuretics; increased risk of GI side effects with drugs having similar side effects such as corticosteroids; potentiation of anticoagulant effects when given with other drugs having same effect; hypoglycemia with insulin; decreased effect of antihypertensives; increased serum lithium levels; not recommended with any other nonsteroidal anti-inflammatory drugs. **Foods:** None	* Assess for prior allergy to aspirin or other nonsteroidal anti-inflammatory drugs. * Patients with asthma at higher risk for allergy. * Assess for visual disturbances and bleeding disorders. * Administration with food may decrease GI discomfort. * Monitor BUN, creatinine, SGOT, SGPT, and serum K+ levels in patients with renal or hepatic dysfunction. * Monitor bleeding time in patients with bleeding disorders. * If visual disturbances occur, eye exam as necessary. * Patient/parent education: - OTC doses are not intended for home management of pain. - Give with food to decrease GI discomfort. - Avoid alcohol and other OTC drugs. - Report rash, flu-like symptoms, visual changes, and/or yellowing of skin.

Name	Uses	Route and Dose	Adverse Reactions/ Side Effects	Drug or Food Interactions	Nursing Considerations
Generic: Lorazepam **Trade:** Ativan	Management of anxiety, provide preoperative sedation and amnesia, status epilepticus.	**Anxiety and sedation:** Infants & children: Oral, IV: 0.05 mg/-0.1 mg/kg/ dose every 4-8 hrs; max 4 mg/dose Adults: 1-10 mg/day in 2-3 divided doses **Insomnia:** Oral: 2 mg at bedtime **Preoperative:** IM: 0.05 mg/kg 2 hrs before surgery, not to exceed 4 mg/dose IV: 0.044 mg/kg 15-20 mins before surgery, not to exceed 4 mg/single dose **Status epilepticus:** IV: Neonates: 0.05 mg/kg over 2-5 mins, may repeat in 10-15 mins Infants & Children: 0.1 mg/kg over 2-5 mins; do not exceed 4 mg/dose; may repeat second dose of 0.05 mg/kg in 10-15 mins if needed Adolescents: 0.07 mg/kg over 2-5 mins; max 4 mg/dose; may repeat 10-15 mins	**CNS:** Drowsiness, sedation, dizziness, weakness, unsteadiness, disorientation, depression, sleep disturbance, restlessness, confusion, hallucinations **CV:** Hyper- or hypotension **GI:** Nausea, vomiting, abdominal discomfort, anorexia **Sensory:** Blurred vision, diplopia, depressed hearing	**Drugs:** Added depressant effects when used with other CNS depressants. **Foods:** None	* Assess vital signs prior to administration. * Assess airway patency prior to IV administration. * Dilute IV doses with an equal volume prior to administration. * Avoid giving this drug intra-arterially as it may lead to gangrene and amputation. * Refrigerate parenteral preparations. * Patient/parent education: - Avoid other OTC medications unless approved by MD. - Instruct patient that amnesia may follow a preoperative dose of this drug. - Avoid alcohol. - Avoid caffeine as it counteracts this drug. * Administer at a rate not to exceed 2 mg/minute.

Name	Uses	Route and Dose	Adverse Reactions/ Side Effects	Drug or Food Interactions	Nursing Considerations
Generic: Meperidine **Trade:** Demerol, Mepergan	Narcotic analgesic used for relief of moderate to severe pain and as a preoperative medication to enhance effects of anesthesia.	Children: Oral, IM, IV, SC: 1-15 mg/kg/dose every 3-4 hrs as needed: max dose 100 mg/dose Sedation/analgesia for procedures: IV: 0.5-1 mg/kg given 2-5 mins before procedure. Adolescents >12 yrs: Sedation/analgesia for procedures: IV: 40 mg, can repeat 1-2 mins at 5 min intervals.	**CNS:** Sedation, dizziness, depression, coma, euphoria, restlessness, insomnia **CV:** Circulatory depression, orthostatic hypotension, palpitation, bradycardia, tachycardia (more common than with other opiates) **GI:** Nausea, vomiting, constipation **Resp:** Respiratory depression **Hepatic:** Biliary spasm, increased serum amylase and lipase **GU:** Urinary retention, oliguria, impotence **Skin:** Rash, erythema, urticaria, pruritus, facial flushing	**Drugs:** Potentiated CNS effects with other CNS depressants; phenothiazines may antagonize action; may potentiate neuro-muscular-blocking agents; may decrease effects of diuretics used in CHF; do not give within 14 days of MAO inhibitors; incompatible with aminophylline, heparin, methicillin, phenobarbital, sodium bicarbonate. **Food:** None	* Assess type and degree of pain. * Baseline vital signs. * Evaluate pain relief/control within 30 minutes of administration. * Patient/parent education: - Take only as directed and only for patient prescribed. - Produces altered mental alertness, therefore, avoid driving and adjust other activities as necessary.

Name	Uses	Route and Dose	Side Effects	Interactions	Considerations
Generic: Midazolam Hydrochloride **Trade:** Versed	Benzodiazepine used to reduce anxiety, as a muscle relaxant, and as an amnesiac. Also used for induction of general anesthesia and to reduce anxiety prior to diagnostic tests such as CT scan.	Infants & Children: Preoperative sedation: Oral:<5 yrs: 0.5 mg/kg >5 yrs: 0.4-0.5 mg/kg, may give up to 0.75 mg/kg/ dose IM: 0.07-0.08 mg/kg 1-2 hrs before surgery IV: 0.035 mg/kg/dose, repeat over several mins as required to achieve the desired sedative effect, up to a total dose of 0.1-0.2 mg/kg Intranasal: 0.2 mg/kg into the nares over 15 secs; may repeat in 5-15 mins Conscious sedation for procedures: Oral: 0.2-0.4 mg/kg (max: 15 mg) 30-45 mins before the procedure Adolescents >12 yrs: Conscious sedation for procedures: IV: 0.5 mg every 3-4 mins until effect achieved.	**CNS:** Excessive sedation, drowsiness, paradoxical excitement, hyperactivity, anxiety, restlessness, confusion **CV:** Hypotension, bradycardia, tachycardia **GI:** Nausea, vomiting, increased salivation, dry mouth, constipation **Resp:** Decreased respiratory rate, apnea **Skin:** Pain at injection site, urticaria, rash, pruritus **Sensory:** Blurred vision, diplopia, nystagmus, blocked ears	**Drugs:** Potentiated with other CNS depressants; potentiated by cimetidine or ranitidine. **Food:** None	* Baseline vital signs. * Provide for patient safety following administration (raise side rails, etc.). * Place patient on cardiac/respiratory monitor if administering IV and have emergency equipment available. * Monitor blood pressure for hypotension. * Monitor for respiratory depression. * Patient/parent education: - Avoid other CNS depressants when taking this medication. * Administer by slow IV push over at least 2 mins at a concentration of 1-5 mg/ml or IV infusion. * Pulse oximeter during administration.

Name	Uses	Route and Dose	Adverse Reactions/ Side Effects	Drug or Food Interactions	Nursing Considerations
Generic: Morphine Sulfate **Trade:** Morphine	Narcotic analgesic used for treatment of severe pain and preoperatively.	Infants & children: Oral: Tablet and solution (prompt release): 0.2-0.5 mg/kg/dose every 4-6 hrs as needed; tablet (controlled release): 0.3-0.6 mg/kg/dose every 12 hrs. IM, IV, SC: 0.1-0.2 mg/kg/dose every 2-4 hrs as needed; max 15 mg/dose IV, SC, continuous infusion: 0.025 mg-2 mg/kg/hour Sedation/analgesia for procedures: IV 0.05-0.1 mg/kg 5 mins before procedure Adolescents >12 yrs: Sedation/analgesia for procedures: IV: 3-4 mg and repeat in 5 mins if necessary	**CNS:** Sedation, coma, dizziness, depression, euphoria, restlessness, insomnia **CV:** Circulatory depression orthostatic hypotension, bradycardia, tachycardia **GI:** Nausea, vomiting, constipation **Resp:** Respiratory depression **Hepatic:** Biliary spasm, increased serum amylase and lipase **GU:** Urinary retention, oliguria, impotence **Skin:** Rash, erythema, urticaria, pruritus, facial flushing	**Drugs:** Potentiated by other CNS depressants; antagonized by phenothiazines; may decreased effects of diuretics in CHF. **Food:** None	* Obtain baseline vital signs, particularly respiratory rate. * Assess type and amount of pain. * Monitor vital signs q 15-30 minutes following administration. * Assess effectiveness 30 minutes following administration. * Have naloxone available to treat side effects (including itching as it is a side effect of the morphine and not histimine related). * Provide for patient safety (side rail up, etc.). * Patient/parent education: - This medication should be used only as directed and only for patient prescribed. - Report any side effects such as itching or nausea and administer naloxone as ordered.

Table 2. ANTIBIOTICS

Name	Uses	Route and Dose	Adverse Reactions/ Side Effects	Drug or Food Interactions	Nursing Considerations
Generic: Amikacin **Trade:** Amikin	Aminoglycoside active against gram + and gram - bacteria used for treatment of infections of bone, burns, urinary tract, and CNS and for septicemia and otitis media.	IV, IM: Neonates: Postnatal age 0-4 weeks, <1200 g: 7.5 mg/kg/dose every 18-24 hrs Postnatal age < or = to 7 days: 1200-2000 g: 7.5 mg/kg/ dose every 12-18 hrs >2000 g: 10 mg/kg/dose every 12 hrs Postnatal age >7 days, 1200-2000 g: 7.5 mg/kg/ dose divided every 8-12 hrs. Infants and children: 15-22.5 mg/kg/day divided every 8 hrs. Adults: 15 mg/kg/day divided every 8-12 hrs	**CNS:** Neurotoxicity, neuromuscular blockade, numbness, tingling, muscle twitching, seizures, lethargy **GI:** Nausea, vomiting, loss of appetite **GU:** Nephrotoxicity, blood in urine, oliguria, proteinuria **Skin:** Rash, drug fever **Hemic:** Eosinophilia, anemia **Sensory:** Ototoxicity	**Drug:** Increased chance of ototoxicity if used with other aminoglycosides and capreomycin. Ototoxicity and nephrotoxicity chances increased if used with Amphotericin B, salicylates, bacitracin (parenteral), bumetanide (parenteral), carmustine, cephalothin, cisplatin, cyclosporine, ethacrynic acid, furosemide, paromomycin, streptozocin, vancomycin. Increases respiratory depressant effects of opioids and analgesics. Inactivated by penicillin, carbicillin, and ticarcillin. **Food:** None	* Culture and sensitivity should be obtained prior to starting treatment. * Do not give IV push. * Do not use solution if it is dark yellow or has particulate matter. * Dilute to maximum amount. * Monitor hearing. * Assess renal function by monitoring I&O, daily weights, urine specific gravity, UA, creatinine levels, and BUN.
Generic: — Amoxicillin — Amoxicillin with Clavulanate potassium **Trade:** Amoxil (without clavulanate potassium) Augmentin (with clavulanate potassium)	Antibiotic used to treat infections of ear, respiratory tract, urinary tract, and skin and soft tissue.	25-50 mg/kg/24 hrs in 3 divided doses Adjust dose in patients with renal impairment.	**GI:** Diarrhea (more common with clavulanate potassium), nausea, vomiting (common with clavulanate potassium), epigastric pain, stomatitis, glossitis **Hepatic:** Moderate rise in SGOT and SGPT **GU:** Superinfections (primarily yeast), interstitial nephritis **Skin:** Erythematous, maculopapular, mildly pruritic rash **Hemic:** Anemia, thrombocytopenia, thrombocytopenic purpura, agranulocytosis, leukopenia, eosinophilia	**Drugs:** Erythromycin, tetracycline, chloromycetin, and acids. Probenecid decreases renal excretion and prolongs serum levels. **Food:** None	* Assess for previous allergy to amoxicillin, penicillin, cephalosporins. * Assess for asthma and family history of allergies. * Monitor for hypersensitivity reaction (first 20 minutes). * Monitor for signs of superinfection. * Patient/parent education: - Finish all medication. - Note any side effects and report to physician. - Reconstituted suspension should be discarded after 14 days.

Name	Uses	Route and Dose	Adverse Reactions/ Side Effects	Drug or Food Interactions	Nursing Considerations

Generic: Ampicillin
 	
Trade: Omnipen Polycillin
	Broad spectrum antibiotic used to treat infections of the ear, meninges, upper respiratory tract, GU tract, skin and soft tissue.	PO:
		50-100 mg/kg/day equally divided q 6h
		
		IV, IM:
		Neonates:
		< 7 days: 50 -100 mg/kg/day divided q 12h
		> 7 days: 100-200 mg/kg/day divided q 8h
		
		Mild - moderate infections:
		50-100 mg/kg/day divided q 6h
		
		Severe infections:
		200-400 mg/kg/day divided q 4-6h
			CNS: Seizures (usually seen in excess of 400 mg/kg/day)
			GI: Diarrhea, nausea, vomiting, epigastric pain, pseudomembranous colitis, stomatitis, glossitis, black tongue
			Hepatic: Moderate rise in SGOT
			GU: Superinfections, primarily yeast
			Skin: Erythematous, maculopapular, mildly pruritus rash
			Hemic: Eosinophilia, anemia, thrombocytopenia, thrombocytopenic purpura, leukopenia, agranulocytosis
				Drugs: Erythromycin, tetracycline, chloramphenicol decrease effects; allopurinol may enhance development of rash; may interfere with effectiveness of oral contraceptives
				
				Food: Absorption hampered by food
					* Assess for previous allergy to drug, penicillins, cephalosporins, other drugs, asthma, or family history of allergies.
					* Obtain culture and sensitivity prior to beginning treatment.
					* Give 1 hr prior or 2 hrs following meals.
					* Reconstitute with sterile or bacteriostatic water .
					* Do not use bacteriostatic preparations containing benzyl alcohol with neonates.
					* Do not exceed IV rate of 100 mg/minute.
					* Stability decreases with dextrose.
					* Observe for signs of hypersensitivity (first 20 min after first dose) or super-infection.
					* Patient/parent education:
					  - Finish all medication.
					  - Monitor for side effects and report rash or diarrhea to physician.
					  - May interfere with effectiveness of oral contraceptives.

Name	Uses	Route and Dose	Adverse Reactions/ Side Effects	Drug or Food Interactions	Nursing Considerations

Generic: Azithromycin
 	
Trade: Zithromax
	Treatment of mild to moderate upper and lower respiratory tract infections, infections of the skin and skin structure, and sexually transmitted diseases due to susceptible strains of *C trachomatis, M. catarrhalis, H. influenzae, S. aureus, S. pneumoniae, Mycoplasma pneumoniae,* and *C. psitacci.*	Oral:
		Children 6 mos and older: Otitis media: 10 mg/kg on day 1 (maximum 500 mg/day) followed by 5 mg/kg/day once daily on days 2-5 (maximum 250 mg/day).
		Children 2 yrs and older: Pharyngitis, tonsillitis: 12 mg/kg/day once daily for 5 days (maximum 500 mg/day).
		Adolescents 16 yrs and older: Respiratory tract, skin and soft tissue infections: 500 mg on day 1 followed by 250 mg/day on days 2-5 (maximum 600 mg/day)
		Uncomplicated chlamydial urethritis or cervicitis: Single 1 G dose.
			CNS: Fever
			Dermatologic: Alopecia, rash
			GI: Nausea, vomiting anorexia, diarrhea, aphthous stomatitis, pancreatitis
			Hematologic: Bone marrow depression (leukopenia, thrombocytopenia, anemia)
			Hepatic: Hepatotoxicity
			Neuromuscular & skeletal: Arthralgias
			Ocular: Retinopathy
			Other: Rare hypersensitive reactions which include myalgias, rigors, maculopapular rash, dyspnea, hypotension.
				Drug: Decreased peak serum levels with aluminum- and magnesium-containing antacids by 24% but not total absorption. Increased effective/toxicity/levels of alfentanil, anticoagulants, astemizole, terfenadine, loratidine, bromocriptine, carbamazepine, cyclosporine, digoxin disopyramide, theophylline, and triazolam.
				
				Food: Presence of food decreases bioavailability by up to 50%.
					* Assess for previous allergy to this drug and to erythromycin, or any macrolide antibiotic.
					* Use with caution in patients with hepatic dysfunction.
					* Obtain culture and sensitivity prior to starting medication if indicated.
					* Patient/parent education:
					  - Finish all medication.
					  - Observe for side effects.
					  - Take on empty stomach 1 hr before meal or 2 hrs after.
					  - Do not take with aluminum- or magnesium-containing antacids.

Generic: Cefaclor
 	
Trade: Ceclor
	Second generation cephalosporin used to treat otitis media, respiratory, urinary tract and skin infections.	PO:
		> 1 mo: 20-40 mg/kg/day divided q 8-12h
			CNS: Headache, dizziness
			GI: Diarrhea, nausea, vomiting, anorexia, cramps, heartburn
			GU: Increased BUN and serum creatinine, vaginitis
			Hemic: Increased SGOT, SGPT, alkaline phosphatase
				Drugs: None noted
				
				Food: Food decreases absorption time.
					* Assess for previous allergy to drug, penicillins, cephalosporins, other drugs, asthma, or family history of allergies.
					* Medication is expensive — use only with susceptible organisms.
					* Monitor for superinfection.
					* Patient/parent education:
					  - Finish all medication.
					  - Observe for side effects.
					  - Store suspension in refrigerator and discard after 14 days.

Name	Uses	Route and Dose	Adverse Reactions/ Side Effects	Drug or Food Interactions	Nursing Considerations
Generic: Cefazolin **Trade:** Kefzol Ancef	First generation cephalosporin used to treat respiratory, biliary and GU tract, skin, bone and joint infections, septicemia, and endocarditis.	IM, IV: < 7 days: 40 mg/kg/day divided q 12h 1 - 4 wks: 60 mg/kg/day divided q 8h > 1 mo: 25-100 mg/kg/day divided q 8h **Maximum dose: 6 g/day** Adjust dose in renal impairment	**GI:** <u>Pseudomembranous colitis</u>, anorexia, diarrhea, thrush, abdominal cramps, nausea, vomiting **GU:** Transient rise in BUN, SGOT, SGPT and alkaline phosphatase, pruritus, genital moniliasis, vaginitis **Hemic:** Transient neutropenia, leukopenia, <u>thrombocytopenia</u>	**Drugs:** Combination with probenecid inhibits renal excretion, thus prolonging serum levels; aminoglycosides, chloramphenicol, and penicillins may cause synergistic effects. **Food:** None	* Assess for previous allergy to cefazolin, cephalosporins, and penicillins. * Obtain culture and sensitivity prior to starting medication. * Monitor for hypersensitivity, symptoms of superinfection, and diarrhea. * IVP.
Generic: Cefotaxime **Trade:** Claforan	Third generation cephalosporin used to treat infections of lower respiratory tract, skin, GU tract, bone, joint, and septicemias, gynecologic, CNS infections, and gonococcal ophthalmic infections.	IV, IM: Neonates: Postnatal age <7 days: 100 mg/kg/24 hrs in 2 divided doses Postnatal age >7 days: 150 mg/kg/24 hrs in 3 divided doses Infants & Children 1 mo to 12 yrs: <50 kg: 100-200 mg/kg/24 hrs in 3-4 divided doses Meningitis: 200 mg/kg/24 hrs in 4 divided doses >50 kg: Moderate to severe infection: 1-2 g every 608 hrs; life threatening infection: 2 g/dose every 4 hrs	**CNS:** Headache **GI:** <u>Pseudomembranous colitis</u>, diarrhea, nausea, vomiting **Hepatic:** Transient rise of SGOT, SGPT, serum LDH, serum alkaline phosphatase **GU:** Transient rise BUN, moniliasis, vaginitis **Skin:** Maculopapular or erythematous rash, pruritus, fever **Hemic:** <u>Granulocytopenia</u>, transient eosinophilia, leukopenia, neutropenia, thrombocytopenia	**Drugs:** Probenecid inhibits renal excretion, thus prolonging serum levels; synergistic effects with certain organisms when combined with aminoglycosides, chloramphenicol, and penicillins; nephrotoxicity increased with concomitant administration of aminoglycosides, potassium-depleting diuretics, and other cephalosporins. **Food:** None	* Assess for previous allergy to cefotaxime, penicillins, or cephalosporins. * Obtain culture and sensitivity prior to starting medication. * IM injection painful. * Do not premix with other aminoglycosides, aminophylline, sodium bicarbonate, or alkaline solutions. * Monitor for hypersensitivity and side effects. * Can be administered IV push over 3-5 mins, or IV retrograde or IV intermittent infusion over 15-30 mins; final concentration for IV administration should not exceed 200 mg/ml.

Name	Uses	Route and Dose	Adverse Reactions/ Side Effects	Drug or Food Interactions	Nursing Considerations
Generic: Clarithromycin **Trade:** Biaxin	Treatment of upper and lower respiratory tract infections, and infections of the skin and skin structure due to susceptible strains of *S. aureus*, *S. pyogenes*, *S. Pneumoniae*, *H. influenzae*, *M. catarrhalis*, *Mycoplasma pneumoniae*, *C. trachomatis*, *Legionella* spp., and *M. avium*.	**Oral:** Children under 6 mos and older: 15 mg/kg/day divided every 12 hrs; dosages of 15-30 mg/kg/day divided every 12 hrs have been used in clinical trials in children with AIDS and disseminated MAC infection.	**GI:** Diarrhea, nausea, vomiting, dyspepsia, abdominal pain (incidence lower than patients treated with erythromycin) **CNS:** Headache **Dermatologic:** Rash, pruritis **Hematologic:** Increased prothrombin time, decreased WBC **Hepatic:** Increased enzymes, hyperbilirubinemia **Renal:** Elevated BUN and creatinine	**Drugs:** Increase serum theophylline levels by as much as 20%; carbamazepine levels have been shown to increase after a single dose of clarithromycin, astemizole; terfenadine; use of clarithromycin and cisapride results in accumulation of an active metabolite of cisapride that is cardiotoxic, increased levels of this metabolite may cause sudden death. **Food:** None.	* Assess for previous allergies to this drug, Erythromycin, or any macrolide antibiotic. * Obtain culture and sensitivity as indicated prior to starting medication. * Reconstituted oral suspension should not be refrigerated because it might gel. * Suspension is stable for 14 days when stored at room temperature. * Patient/parent education: - Finish all medication - Observe for any side effects - Store at room temperature

Name	Uses	Route and Dose	Adverse Reactions/ Side Effects	Drug or Food Interactions	Nursing Considerations
Generic: Clindamycin **Trade:** Cleocin	Antibiotic useful against aerobic and anaerobic streptococci (except enterococci), most staphylococci, used topically in treatment of severe acne.	**Neonates: IV, IM:** Postnatal age <7 days: <2000 g: 10 mg/kg/24 hrs divided every 12 hrs >2000 g: 15 mg/kg/24 hrs divided every 8 hrs Postnatal age > days: <2000 g: 15 mg/kg/24 hrs divided every 9 hrs >2000 g: 20 mg/kg/24 hrs divided every 6-8 hrs **Infants & Children:** Oral: 10-30 mg/kg/24 hrs in 3-4 divided doses IV, IM: 25-40 mg/kg/24 hrs divided every 6-8 hrs Children and adults topical: Apply twice daily **Adults:** Oral: 150-450 mg/kg/dose every 6-8 hrs; maximum dose: 1.8 g/day IV, IM: 600-1200 mg/24 hrs in 2-4 divided doses.	**GI:** Pseudomembranous colitis, diarrhea, nausea, vomiting, abdominal pain, flatulence, esophagitis **Hepatic:** Transient rise of SGOT, serum bilirubin, alkaline phosphatase **GU:** Azotemia, oliguria, proteinuria **Skin:** Topical: dryness, erythema, burning, peeling, pruritus **Hemic:** Transient leukopenia, neutropenia, thrombocytopenia, eosinophilia, agranulocytosis **Musculoskeletal:** Polyarthritis **Other:** Hypersensitivity (maculopapular rash, urticaria, pruritus erythema multiforme); local: IM - pain, induration, sterile abscess; IV - pain, edema, erythema, thrombophlebitis, hypotension and cardiac arrest if infused too rapidly	**Drugs:** May potentiate neuromuscular blocking agents such as pancuronium and atracurium, possible antagonism with aminoglycosides **Foods:** None	* Assess for previous allergy to this drug or lincomycin. * Obtain culture and sensitivity prior to starting medication. * Obtain baseline hematological, renal, and hepatic studies prior to beginning long-term therapy. * Observe and report appearance of skin with topical use. * Do not refrigerate po solutions. * May give with food. * If given PO, encourage fluids to avoid esophagitis. * IM injection is painful — do not give 600 mg per injection site. * Do not give IV push. * Dilute IV doses to a minimum of 6 mg/ml and give no faster than 30 mg/minute. * Avoid eye area with topical applications. * Monitor IM injection sites for induration and abscess. * Monitor IV sites for extravasation and thrombophlebitis. * Monitor for superinfection, primarily yeast. * Patient/parent education: - Teach proper application of topical solution. - Emphasize strict adherence to oral dosing schedule. - Stress need for continued close medical supervision during therapy. - Report any adverse reactions (especially diarrhea) to MD.

Name	Uses	Route and Dose	Adverse Reactions/ Side Effects	Drug or Food Interactions	Nursing Considerations
Generic: Dicloxacillin sodium **Trade:** Dynapen	Antibiotic that is the drug of choice for oral use in treating penicillinase-producing *Staphylococcus aureus* and *S. epidermidis* infections.	**PO:** > 1 mo: < 40 kg: 12.5-25 mg/kg/day equally divided q 6h > 40 kg: 125-500 mg every 6 hrs	**GI:** Nausea, vomiting, epigastric pain, loose stools, diarrhea, flatulence, hemorrhagic colitis **Hepatic:** Transient rise in SGOT, SGPT **Skin:** Rashes, pruritus indicating hypersensitivity **Hemic:** Eosinophilia, anemia, neutropenia, thrombocytopenia, leukopenia **Other:** Hypersensitivity indicated by drug fever	**Drugs:** Erythromycin, tetracycline, chloromycetin decrease antibacterial effects. **Food:** Food interferes with absorption of this medication.	* Assess for previous allergy to drug, penicillins, cephalosporins, other drugs, asthma, other allergies. * Obtain culture and sensitivity prior to starting medication. * Give on empty stomach (1 hour prior or 2 hours following meals) as food interferes with absorption. * Refrigerate solution and shake well. * Monitor for hypersensitivity, rash, and other side effects. * Maintain fluid intake. * Patient/parent education: - Finish all medication. - Observe for side effects such as diarrhea. - Do not take OTC drugs without consulting MD. - Store solution in refrigerator out of reach of children and discard after 14 days.

Name	Uses	Route and Dose	Adverse Reactions/ Side Effects	Drug or Food Interactions	Nursing Considerations
Generic: Erythromycin **Trade:** E-Mycin **Generic:** Erythromycin ethylsuccinate **Trade:** E.E.S. Pediamycin **Generic:** Erythromycin estolate **Trade:** Ilosone	Antibiotic active against gram + and – bacteria used to treat infections of respiratory tract, skin, soft tissue, otitis media, Lyme disease, neonatal conjunctivitis and ocular infections, acne and superficial wounds.	Newborns: Oral: 20-30 mg/kg/24 hrs divided every 8-12 hrs Children: Oral: 30-50 mg/kg/24 hrs in 4 divided doses every 6 hrs; max daily dose 1-2 g IV: 20-40 mg/kg/24 hrs as a continuous IV infusion (every 6 hrs in divided doses by intermittent IV infusion; maximum 2-4 g/day) Ophthalmic: Prophylaxis neonatal gonococcal ophthalmia: Instill 0.5 - 2 cm strip into conjunctival sac within 1 hour post delivery Combination form: Pediazole: > 2 months: 50 mg erythromycin and 150 mg sulfisoxazole/kg/day equally divided q 6h	**GI:** Abdominal pain and cramping, nausea, vomiting, diarrhea, stomatitis, anorexia **Skin:** Dryness, erythema, burning, peeling **Sensory:** Tinnitus, vertigo, ototoxicity, reversible bilateral hearing loss **Other:** Anaphylaxis, urticaria, skin eruptions, rash **Local:** IV: Venous irritation, thrombophlebitis; IM causes severe pain	**Drugs:** Antagonistic action if given with clindamycin; potential toxicity if given with carbamazepine, cyclosporine, theophylline, and digoxin; increased effects if given with oral anticoagulants. **Foods:** Absorption delayed if administered with food depending upon formulation prescribed.	* Assess for previous allergy. * Obtain culture and sensitivity prior to starting medication. * Give on empty stomach. * Do not crush film or enteric-coated tablets. * May take apart time release capsules but instruct patient not to chew particles. * Do not give IV push or rapid infusion * Give IV solution slowly as solution is irritating. * Observe for adverse reactions/side effects. * Patient/parent education: - Finish all medication. - Observe for side effects. - Teach proper administration technique.

Name	Uses	Route and Dose	Adverse Reactions/ Side Effects	Drug or Food Interactions	Nursing Considerations
Generic: Erythromycin and Sulfisoxazole **Trade:** Pediazole	Treatment of susceptible bacterial infections of the upper and lower respiratory tract; otitis media, other infections in patients allergic to penicillin.	Dosage recommendation based on the product's erythromycin content. Children 2 mos of age and older: Oral: 40-50 mg/kg/24 hrs in divided doses every 6 hrs; not to exceed 2 g erythromycin or 6 g sulfisoxazole every 24 hrs	**CNS:** Headache, lethargy, nervousness, ataxia, mental depression, seizures, hallucinations **GI:** Nausea, vomiting, diarrhea, GI pain, stomatitis, pseudomembranous enterocolitis, pancreatitis **Hepatic:** Jaundice **GU:** Crystalluria, increased BUN and serum creatinine, oliguria, hematuria, proteinuria **Hemic:** Granulocytopenia, agranulocytosis, thrombocytopenia, leukopenia, hemolytic anemia, aplastic anemia, neutropenia **Other:** Epidermal necrolysis, Stevens-Johnson syndrome, exfoliative dermatitis, allergic myocarditis, serum sickness, anaphylaxis	**Drugs:** Theophylline, carbamazepine, cyclosporine, triazolam; risk of serious cardiac arrhythmias exists in patients receiving erythromycin and astemizole or terfenadine; cisapride. **Food:** Decreased absorption if given with food but may do so if nausea occurs.	* Assess for previous allergy to drug combination or sulfonamides. * Obtain culture and sensitivity prior to starting medication. * Assess baseline CBC, UA, renal function tests, especially if treatment > 2 weeks. * May be mixed or given with food if gastric distress noted. * Maintain hydration to prevent crystalluria. * Assess for sore throat, fever, skin rash, and sore mouth and signs of blood dyscrasias. * Patient/parent education: - Finish all medication as prescribed. - Observe for side effects. - Teach proper administration technique. - Maintain hydration levels. - Protect child from sun. - Store suspension at room temperature. - Consult MD prior to taking OTC medications.

Name	Uses	Route and Dose	Adverse Reactions/ Side Effects	Drug or Food Interactions	Nursing Considerations
Generic: Gentamycin **Trade:** Garamycin	Aminoglycoside active against wide range of gram + and - bacteria. Used to treat infections of bone, skin, urinary and GI tract, neonatal and bacterial septicemias, meningitis, external eye and adnexa, primary and secondary skin infections.	Dosage should be based on body weight. Neonates: IM, IV: Postnatal age <7 days: <1000 g and <28 weeks GA: 2.5 mg/kg/dose every 24 hrs <1500 g and <34 weeks GA: 2.5 mg/kg/dose every 18 hrs >1500 g and >34 weeks GA: 2.5 mg/kg/dose every 12 hrs Postnatal age >7 days: <2000 g: 2.5 mg/kg/dose every 12 hrs >2000 g: 2.5 mg/kg/dose every 8 hrs Infants & Children: Oral: For bacterial overgrowth of the intestinal tract: 10-30 mg/kg/24 hrs divided every 8 hrs IM, IV: 2.5 mg/kg/dose every 8 hrs Topical: Apply 3-4 times/ day Ophthalamic: Solution: 1-2 drops every 2-4 hrs up to 2 drops/hr for severe infections; Ointment: 2-3 times/day Intrathecal: Newborns: 1 mg/day Infants >3 mos and children: 1-2 g/day	**CNS:** Neurotoxicity, neuromuscular blockade, numbness, tingling, muscle twitching and weakness, respiratory depression, lethargy, headache **GI:** Nausea, vomiting, loss of appetite **GU:** Nephrotoxicity, increased BUN and creatinine, oliguria, renal failure **Skin:** Itching, redness, edema **Hemic:** Agranulocytosis, anemia, leukopenia, eosinophilia, thrombocytopenia **Sensory:** Ototoxicity, hearing loss due to damage to eighth cranial nerve, tinnitus	**Drugs:** Increased chance of ototoxicity and nephrotoxicity if used concurrently with amphotericin B, salicylates, parenteral bacitracin, antineoplastics, vancomycin; masked symptoms of ototoxicity if used with dimenhydrinate; increased chance of ototoxicity if used with other aminoglycosides; increased respiratory depressant effects of opioids and analgesics, inactivated by parenteral carbenicillin and ticarcillin. **Food:** None	* Assess for previous allergy. * Obtain culture and sensitivity prior to starting medication. * Obtain baseline weights, BUN and creatinine, and hearing tests. * Do not give IV push or rapid infusion. * Observe for adverse reactions/side effects. * Discontinue therapy if no improvement in 3-5 days. * Monitor hearing function. * Patient/parent education: - Finish all medication. - Observe for side effects, including hearing loss. - Teach proper administration technique. - If no improvement in 3-5 days, notify MD. * Obtain drug levels after the third dose. * Administer by IV slow intermittent or retrograde infusion over 3 mins, final concentration for administration should not exceed 40 mg/ml.

Name	Uses	Route and Dose	Adverse Reactions/ Side Effects	Drug or Food Interactions	Nursing Considerations
Generic: Kanamycin **Trade:** Kantrex	Aminoglycoside used to treat infections of bone, skin, urinary and GI tract and as preoperative agent for bowel surgery.	PO,IM,IV: **Birth-7 days, ≤ 2000 gm:** 7.5 mg/kg q 12h **Birth-7 days, > 2000 gm:** 7.5 mg/kg q 8 - 12h **1-4 weeks, ≤ 2000 gm:** 10 mg/kg q 12h **1-4 weeks, > 2000 gm:** 10 mg/kg q 8h **> 4 weeks:** 15-30 mg/kg/ day equally divided q 8-12h	**CNS:** Neurotoxicity, neuromuscular blockade, numbness, tingling, muscle twitching and weakness, respiratory depression, lethargy, headache **GI:** Nausea, vomiting, loss of appetite, malabsorption syndrome (long-term therapy) **GU:** Nephrotoxicity, increased BUN and creatinine, oliguria, renal failure **Skin:** Itching, redness, edema **Hemic:** Agranulocytosis, anemia, leukopenia, eosinophilia, thrombocytopenia **Sensory:** Ototoxicity, hearing loss due to damage to eighth cranial nerve, tinnitus	**Drugs:** Increased chance of ototoxicity and nephrotoxicity if used concurrently with amphotericin B, salicylates, parenteral bacitracin, antineoplastics, vancomycin; masked symptoms of ototoxicity if used with dimenhydrinate; increased chance of ototoxicity if used with other aminoglycosides; increased respiratory depressant effects of opioids and analgesics, inactivated by parenteral penicillin, carbenicillin and ticarcillin. **Food:** None	* Assess for previous allergy. * Obtain culture and sensitivity prior to starting medication. * Obtain baseline weights, BUN and creatinine, and hearing tests. * Solution may darken with age without affecting potency. * May mix with food. * If used prior to bowel surgery, dose same as for adults. * Do not give IV push or rapid infusion. * Monitor blood levels of medication. * Observe for adverse reactions/side effects. * Discontinue therapy if no improvement in 3-5 days. * Monitor hearing function. * Patient/parent education: - Finish all medication. - Observe for side effects, including hearing loss. - Teach proper administration technique. - If no improvement in 3-5 days, notify MD.

Name	Uses	Route and Dose	Adverse Reactions/ Side Effects	Drug or Food Interactions	Nursing Considerations
Generic: Nafcillin **Trade:** Nafcil Unipen	Antibiotic used for penicillinase-producing *Staphylococcus aureus* and *S. epidermidis* infections.	**Neonates:** IM, IV: Mild to moderate infections: Postnatal age <7 days; <2000 g: 50 mg/kg/24 hrs in divided doses every 12 hrs; >2000 g: 75 mg/kg/24 hrs in divided doses every 6-8 hrs **Severe infections:** Postnatal age <7 days: 100 mg/kg/24 hrs in divided doses every 8-12 hrs Postnatal age >7 days: 150 mg/kg/24 hrs in divided doses every 6-8 hrs **Children:** IM-IV: Mild to moderate infections: 50-100 mg/kg/24 hrs in divided doses every 6 hrs Severe infections: 100-200 mg/kg/24 hrs in divided doses every 4-6 hrs Max dose: 12 g/24 hrs	**GI:** Nausea, vomiting, diarrhea **GU:** Hematuria, dysuria, oliguria, proteinuria **Hepatic:** Transient rise in SGOT, SGPT, alkaline phosphatase **Skin:** Rashes, pruritus **Hemic:** <u>Agranulocytosis,</u> anemia, <u>leukopenia,</u> <u>eosinophilia,</u> <u>thrombocytopenia,</u> <u>neutropenia</u> **Other:** <u>Serum sickness,</u> <u>anaphylaxis</u> **Local:** IM painful, sterile abscesses, IV: phlebitis, thrombophlebitis, <u>extra-</u> <u>vasation causes severe</u> <u>chemical irritation that can</u> <u>result in full thickness skin</u> <u>loss and gangrene</u>	**Drugs:** Erythromycin, tetracycline, chloramphenicol decrease antibacterial effects; potentiates anticoagulants; serum concentrations increased and half-life prolonged by probenecid. **Food:** Interferes with absorption; give on empty stomach.	* Assess for previous allergy to this drug, penicillins, cephalosporins, other drugs, asthma and family history of allergies. * Obtain culture and sensitivity prior to starting medication. * Obtain baseline renal, hepatic, and hematologic tests. * Administer on empty stomach. * Injection is painful. * Monitor carefully if given IV — extravasation causes severe damage to skin and surrounding tissues. * May give slow IV push. * Monitor IM injection sites for sterile abscess. * Observe for adverse reactions/side effects. * Patient/parent education: - Finish all medication. - Observe for side effects. - Teach proper administration technique.

Name	Uses	Route and Dose	Adverse Reactions/ Side Effects	Drug or Food Interactions	Nursing Considerations
Generic: Nitrofurantoin **Trade:** Macrodantin Furadantin Furan	Anti-infective used primarily in UTI or prophylaxis against UTI.	**PO:** > 1 mo: 5-7 mg/kg/day equally divided q 6 hrs **Prophylaxis: 1-2** mg/kg/day HS or BID	**CNS:** Peripheral neuropathy, headache, vertigo **GI:** Anorexia, nausea, vomiting, abdominal pain and diarrhea **Resp:** Hypersensitivity: 3 types: a) acute: severe dyspnea, chills, fever, cough, chest pain — may occur 8 hrs to 3 weeks after initiation of therapy but reversible if drug stopped; b) subacute: tachypnea, dyspnea, fever, cough — occurs 1 month after initiation of therapy but recovery slower; c) chronic: dyspnea on exertion, altered pulmonary function, malaise, cough — occurs after continuous therapy for 6 months and may cause permanent pulmonary damage **Hepatic:** Cholestatic jaundice, hepatic necrosis **GU:** Dark yellow or brown urine, crystalluria **Skin:** Erythema multiforme, exfoliative dermatitis, Stevens-Johnson syndrome, photosensitivity, transient alopecia **Hemic:** Agranulocytosis, leukopenia, eosinophilia, hemolytic anemia **Other:** Hypersensitivity, asthma (if previous history), anaphylaxis	**Drugs:** Renal excretion impaired and toxicity increased by probenecid and sulfinpyrazone; magnesium trisilicate antacids decrease absorption; antagonizes quinolone-derivative anti-infectives. **Food:** None	* Assess for previous allergy. * Obtain culture and sensitivity prior to starting medication. * Assess renal function. * May be mixed or given with food. * Contact with teeth may cause yellow staining. * Maintain hydration. * Observe for adverse reactions/side effects—these are not dose related. * Patient/parent education: - Finish all medication. - Observe for side effects. - Teach proper administration technique. - Inform of discoloration of urine. - Stop medication and inform MD if tingling, numbness, or dyspnea occurs.

Name	Uses	Route and Dose	Adverse Reactions/ Side Effects	Drug or Food Interactions	Nursing Considerations

Generic: Rifampin
 	
Trade: Rifamate
	Antibiotic used to treat *Mycobacterium tuberculosis*, *Neisseria meningitidis*, and for prophylaxis against *Haemophilus Influenzae* type B.	**PO:**
		Antituberculosis:
		5 yrs: 10-20 mg/kg/day
		
		Meningococcal prophylaxis:
		<1 mo: 5 mg/kg/24 hrs in divided doses every 12 hrs for 2 days
		1 mo and older: 10 mg/kg/24 hrs in divided doses every 12 hrs for 2 days
		Infants & children: 20 mg/kg/24 hrs in divided doses every 12 hrs for 2 days
		Adults: 600 mg every 12 hrs for 2 days
		
		Haemophilus Influenzae type B prophylaxis:
		0-1 mo: 10 mg/kg/day QD x 4 days
		>1 mo: 20 mg/kg/day QD x 4 days
		
		Maximum dose: 600 mg/kg/day
			CNS: Headache, fatigue, drowsiness, ataxia, dizziness, confusion, generalized numbness
			GI: Heartburn, epigastric distress, nausea, vomiting, anorexia, diarrhea, flatulence, sore mouth and tongue
			Hepatic: Transient rise in SGPT, SGOT, alkaline phosphatase, bilirubin, jaundice
			GU: Hematuria, hemoglobinuria, increased BUN and serum uric acid, renal insufficiency
			Hemic: Thrombocytopenia, leukopenia, purpura, hemolytic anemia
			Musculoskeletal: Muscle weakness, joint and extremity pain
			Other: Reddish orange color to urine, feces, saliva, sweat and tears; hypersensitivity reaction has flu-like symptoms
				Drug: Increased chance of hepatotoxicity with alcohol intake; causes liver enzymes to inactivate barbiturates, corticosteroids, digitalis derivatives, quinidine, dapsone, cyclosporine, chloramphenicol, oral anticoagulants, estrogens, and oral contraceptives; decreased absorption with concurrent administration of clofazimine.
				
				Food: Absorption may be decreased with food intake but may give with food if gastric distress.
					* Obtain culture and sensitivity prior to starting medication.
					* Assess baseline renal and hematopoietic status.
					* May be mixed or given with food if gastric distress noted.
					* Maintain hydration.
					* Assess for jaundice and other side effects.
					* Patient/parent education:
					  - Finish all medication as prescribed.
					  - Observe for side effects.
					  - Teach proper administration technique.
					  - Inform of discoloration of body fluids.
					  - May permanently discolor contact lens.
					  - Maintain close medical follow-up.

Name	Uses	Route and Dose	Adverse Reactions/ Side Effects	Drug or Food Interactions	Nursing Considerations
Generic: Sulfamethoxazole and Trimethoprim **Trade:** Bactrim	Oral treatment of urinary tract infections, acute otitis media; prophylaxis of Pneumocystis carinii pneumonitis (PCP); IV treatment of documented PCP; treatment of documented or suspected shigellosis, typhoid fever	Children >2 mos: Minor infection: 6-10 mg TMP/kg/24 hrs in divided doses every 12 hrs. Serious infection/ Pneumocystis: 15-20 mg TMP/kg/24 hrs in divided doses every 6 hrs. UTI prophylaxis: 2 mg TMP/kg/dose daily Prophylaxis of Pneumocystis: 5-10 mg TMP/kg/24 hrs	**CNS:** Headache, lethargy, ataxia, nervousness **GI:** Nausea, vomiting, pain, stomatitis, pseudo-membranous enterocolitis, pancreatitis **Hepatic:** Hepatitis **GU:** Increased BUN and creatinine, crystalluria **Skin:** Erythematous, maculopapular, morbilliform rashes, urticaria **Hemic:** Agranulocytosis, aplastic anemia, leukopenia, neutropenia, thrombocytopenia, hemolytic anemia **Other:** Epidermal necrolysis, Steven-Johnson syndrome, exfoliative dermatitis, allergic myocarditis, anaphylaxis	**Drugs:** Use with warfarin may prolong prothrombin time; may displace methotrexate binding sites when used in combination; interferes with bactericidal effects of penicillins; may interfere with hepatic metabolism of phenytoin. **Foods:** May slightly delay absorption — give on empty stomach.	* Assess for previous allergy to sulfonamides. * Obtain culture and sensitivity prior to starting medication. * Give on empty stomach, if possible. * Do not give IV push or rapid infusion * Keep well hydrated. * Observe for adverse reactions/side effects. * Patient/parent education: - Finish all medication. - Observe for side effects. - Maintain hydration. - Protect from sun as this may cause a hypersensitivity reaction. * Infuse over 60-90 mins; must be further diluted (5 ml drug to 125 ml diluent like D5W); in patients who require fluid restriction, a dilution can be administered (5 ml drug to 75 ml diluent like D5W); must be used within 2 hrs after dilution in D5W.

Name	Uses	Route and Dose	Adverse Reactions/ Side Effects	Drug or Food Interactions	Nursing Considerations
Generic: Tetracycline **Trade:** Panmycin Tetraclor	Anti-infective active against a variety of gram + and - organisms although a high percentage (10-40%) of gram - organisms are resistant to the drug.	**PO:** **Older infants and children:** 25-50 mg/kg/day equally divided q 6 hrs **Chlamydia genital infections:** 500 mg q 6 hrs	**CNS:** Dizziness, vertigo, ataxia, drowsiness, fatigue, increased intracranial pressure and bulging fontanel in infants **CV:** Pericarditis **GI:** Nausea, vomiting, diarrhea, epigastric distress, stomatitis, glossitis, dysphagia, black hair tongue, esophageal ulceration, oral candidiasis, pseudomembranous colitis, staphylococcal enterocolitis **Hepatic:** Hepatotoxicity **GU:** Vaginal candidiasis, increased BUN **Hemic:** Leukocytosis, neutropenia, eosinophilia **Other:** Skeletal retardation and tooth staining in young children	**Drugs:** Chelates with divalent or trivalent cations (drugs containing aluminum, calcium, magnesium, iron, zinc); may potentiate oral anticoagulants; fatal toxicity if used with methoxyflurane anesthesia. **Food:** None	* Obtain baseline renal, hepatic, and hematologic studies if long-term therapy. * Obtain culture and sensitivity prior to starting medication. * Check expiration date — outdated medication may cause nephrotoxicity. * Give on empty stomach as food decreases absorption by 50%. * May cause esophageal irritation so do not administer at bedtime to children with reflux and follow with plenty of water. * Patient/parent education: - Finish all medication as prescribed. - Observe for side effects such as superinfection. - Teach proper administration technique. - Protect child from sun.

Name	Uses	Route and Dose	Adverse Reactions/ Side Effects	Drug or Food Interactions	Nursing Considerations
Generic: Ticarcillin **Trade:** Ticar Ticarcipen	Penicillin used to treat infections of the GU and respiratory tracts, intra-abdominal, skin and soft tissue infections, and septicemia and meningitis.	**IV:** **Neonates < 2 kg:** ≤ 7 days: 150 mg/kg/day equally divided q 12h > 7 days: 225 mg/kg/day equally divided q 8h **Neonates > 2 kg:** ≤ 7 days: 225 mg/kg/day equally divided q 8h > 7 days: 300 mg/kg/day equally divided q 6h **Children and adults:** 200-300 mg/kg/day equally divided q 4-6h	**CNS:** Neuromuscular irritability, seizures with high serum levels **GI:** Nausea, vomiting, abnormal taste, flatulence, loose stools, diarrhea **Hepatic:** Elevation of SGOT, SGPT, LDH, alkaline phosphatase, bilirubin **Hemic:** Anemia, eosinophilia, thrombocytopenia, leukopenia, neutropenia, abnormal PTT and clotting time (with high doses) **Other:** Skin rashes, pruritus, urticaria, drug fever, hypernatremia, hypokalemia **Local:** IV administration - pain, venous irritation, phlebitis; IM administration — pain induration	**Drugs:** Increased risk of bleeding with anticoagulants; decreased effects with erythromycin, tetracycline, and chloromycetin; decreased serum levels with probenecid. **Foods:** None	* Assess for previous allergy to this drug, penicillins, cephalosporins, other drugs, and history of other allergies. * Obtain culture and sensitivity prior to starting medication. * Obtain baseline renal, hepatic, hematologic studies and potassium levels if therapy is to be long-term. * By IV intermittent infusion over 30-120 mins or less are preferred to avoid vein irritation. * Monitor for hypersensitivity (especially in first 20 minutes following first administration). * Monitor potassium and sodium levels as well as renal and hepatic function. * Monitor platelets and PTT if on long-term therapy. * Maintain appropriate fluid levels for weight.

Name	Uses	Route and Dose	Adverse Reactions/ Side Effects	Drug or Food Interactions	Nursing Considerations
Generic: Tobramycin **Trade:** Tobrex	Aminoglycoside used to treat known or suspected *Pseudomonas aeruginosa* infection; infection with nonpseudomonal enteric bacillus which is more sensitive to tobramycin than gentamicin based on susceptibility tests; empiric therapy in cystic fibrosis and immunocompromised patients.	IM,IV: Neonates ≤ 7 days: < 28 weeks: 2.5 mg/kg q 24h 28-34 weeks: 2.5 mg/kg q 18h Term: 2.5 mg/kg q 12h Neonates >7 days: < 28 weeks: 2.5 mg/kg q 18h 28-34 weeks: 2.5 mg/kg q 12h Infants, 7 days-1 year: 2.5 mg/kg q 8h > 1 year: 2-2.5 mg/kg q 8h	CNS: Neurotoxicity, neuro-muscular blockade, numb-ness, tingling, muscle twitching and weakness, respiratory depression, lethargy, headache GI: Nausea, vomiting, loss of appetite Hepatic: Increased bilirubin, SGOT, SGPT, hepatomegaly, hepatic necrosis GU: Nephrotoxicity, increased BUN and serum creatinine, decreased urine creatinine clearance and specific gravity, renal failure Skin: Rash, burning, edema Hemic: Agranulocytosis, anemia, leukopenia, eosinophilia, thrombocytopenia Sensory: Ototoxicity, hearing loss due to damage to eighth cranial nerve, cochlear damage indicated by high frequency hearing loss	Drugs: Increased chance of ototoxicity and nephro-toxicity if used concurrently with amphotericin B, salicylates, parenteral bacitracin, antineoplastics, vancomycin; masked symptoms of ototoxicity if used with dimenhydrinate; increased chance of ototoxicity if used with other aminoglycosides; increased effects of opioids and analgesics, inactivated by parenteral carbenicillin and ticarcillin. Foods: None	* Obtain culture and sensitivity prior to starting medication. * Obtain baseline weights, BUN and creatinine, and hearing tests. * Do not infuse in less than 30 mins. * Monitor for signs of respiratory depression during IV infusion. * Do not give IV push or rapid infusion. * Monitor blood levels of medication. * Observe for adverse reactions/side effects. * Discontinue therapy if no improve-ment in 3-5 days. * Monitor hearing function. * Patient/parent education: - Finish all medication. - Observe for side effects, including hearing loss. - Teach proper administration tech-nique. - If no improvement in 3-5 days, notify MD. - If using ointment for ocular infec-tion, do not share towels, wash-cloths, pillow cases, make-up, or the medication with others. - Do not wear contact lens if using eye medication.

Name	Uses	Route and Dose	Adverse Reactions/ Side Effects	Drug or Food Interactions	Nursing Considerations
Generic: Vancomycin **Trade:** Vancocin	Treatment of infections due to documented or suspected methicillin-resistant S. aureus or beta-lactam resistant coagulase negative Stephylococcus; treatment of penicillin resistant, cephalosporin resistant S. Pneumoniae infections.	Neonates: Postnatal age 0-7 days: <1000 g: 10 mg/kg every 24 hrs 1000-2000g: 10 mg/kg every 18 hrs >2000 g: 10 mg/kg every 12 hrs Infants: Postnatal age >7 days: <1000 g: 10 mg/kg every 18 hrs 1000-2000 g: 10 mg/kg every 12 hrs >2000 g: 10 mg/kg every 8 hrs Older infants & children: 30-45 mg/kg/24 hrs divided every 6-8 hrs Endocarditis prophylaxis undergoing dental procedures: IV: Children <27 kg: 20 mg/kg 1 hr before procedure; dose may be repeated in 8-12 hrs in high risk patients Children >27 kg & adults: 1 g 1 hr before procedure; may repeat dose in 8-12 hrs in high risk patients. Antibiotic associated pseudomembranous and staphylococcus enterocolitis: Oral: Neonates: 10 mg/kg/ 24 hrs divided every 6-8 hrs Children: 10 mg/kg/dose every 6 hrs; do not exceed 2 g/24 hrs	Rapid infusion associated with red neck or red man syndrome: Erythema multiforme-like reaction with intense pruritus, tachycardia, hypotension, rash involving face, neck, upper trunk, back and upper arms. **Cardiovascular:** cardiac arrest. **Central nervous system:** Fever, chils. **Dermatologic:** Red neck or red man syndrome, urticaria, macular skin rash. **Gastrointestinal:** Nausea. **Hematologic:** Neutropenia, eosinophilia. **Local:** Phlebitis. **Neuromuscular and skeletal:** Lower back pain. **Otis:** Ototoxicity associated with prolonged serum concentration >40 mcg/ml. **Renal:** Nephrotoxicity. **Miscellaneous:** Hypersensitivity reactions.	Drug: Aesthetic agents. Foods: None.	* Obtain culture and sensitivity prior to starting medication. * Obtain renal function tests, BUN and creatinine, hematological tests and hearing tests. * Infuse over 60 minutes. * Assure patency of IV catheter prior to IV infusion as extravasation causes tissue necrosis . * Do not give IM, IV push, or rapid infusion. * Do not mix with other drugs. * Monitor blood levels of medication. * Monitor hearing function. * Patient/parent education: - Finish all medication. - Observe for side effects, including hearing loss. - Maintain good oral hygiene. - Do not take OTC medications without consulting MD. * Monitor for adverse reactions/side effects, especially red man syndrome, tinnitis.

Table 3. ANTIFUNGALS

Name	Uses	Route and Dose	Adverse Reactions/ Side Effects	Drug or Food Interactions	Nursing Considerations
Generic: Amphotericin B Trade: Fungizone	Antifungal used to treat serious and potentially fatal fungal infections.	Topical: Apply BID - QID IV: (Mix with D₅W to a concentration of 0.1 mg/ml and pH > 4.2) Test dose: 0.1 mg/kg/dose to a maximum of 1 mg; infuse over 30-60 mins. If the test dose is tolerated, give the remainder of the dose over 4-6 hrs. Maintenance dose: 0.5 to 1 mg/kg/24 hrs given once daily; infuse over 6 hrs; once therapy has been established, amphotericin B can be administered on an every other day basis at 1-1.5 mg/kg/dose.	CNS: Headache, peripheral nerve pain, paresthesia, vision changes, arachnoiditis GI: Anorexia, weight loss, dyspepsia, epigastric pain, nausea, vomiting GU: Hypokalemia (80% of patients), hyposthenuria, azotemia, renal tubular acidosis, nephrocalcinosis, permanent renal impairment, anuria, oliguria Hemic: Leukopenia, eosinophilia, thrombocytopenia, agranulocytosis, reversible normocytic, normochromic anemia Skin: Lotion–pruritus, exacerbation of preexisting candidal lesions; cream — drying effect, erythema, burning contact dermatitis Musculoskeletal: Muscle weakness, muscle and joint pain Other: Febrile reaction to IV administration, fever and chills 1-2 hrs after starting IV infusion, pain at infusion site, phlebitis, thrombophlebitis	Drugs: Increased incidence of nephrotoxicity when given with other drugs with the same side effect; enhanced potassium loss if given with cortico-steroids, cardiac glycosides, or skeletal muscle relaxants; use with caution with antineoplastic drugs. Foods: None	* Obtain positive identification of organism prior to starting treatment with this drug. * Obtain baseline BUN, serum creatinine, liver function tests, hematologic tests, and weight. * Do not use reconstituted medication if not clear of precipitate and/or foreign matter. * Do not mix with other medications. * Infuse very slowly (usually over 6 hours). * Obtain full sets of vital signs (including temperature) q 30 mins during infusion. * Monitor for cardiovascular collapse. * Assess I&O, weight, potassium, magnesium, BUN, serum creatinine, bilirubin, alkaline phosphatase, and SGOT QD until routine dose established then q week. * Obtain weekly CBC. * Monitor for signs of hypokalemia. * Patient/parent education: - Teach proper application of topical medications. - If no improvement noted in 2 wks, contact MD. - Treatment may last several months. - May stain clothing. - Remove lotion from hands with soap and warm water. - Remove ointment from hands with cleaning fluid. - Do not apply OTC medications over infected area without con-sulting MD.

Name	Uses	Route and Dose	Adverse Reactions / Side Effects	Drug or Food Interactions	Nursing Considerations

Generic: Griseofulvin
 	
Trade: Fulvicin-U/F
	Antifungal	**PO:**
		> 2 years: 15 - 20 mg/kg/day
			CNS: Headache (early in therapy), fatigue, dizziness, insomnia
			GI: Nausea, vomiting, epigastric distress, polydipsia, flatulence, diarrhea, oral thrush
			Skin: Photosensitivity, urticaria, rashes, angioedema, serumlike sickness
			Hemic: Leukopenia
			Other: Estrogenlike effects, lupus erythematosus or lupuslike syndromes
				Drugs: Flushing and tachycardia with concurrent ingestion of alcohol; decreased drug concentrations with phenobarbital; decrease in PTT if given with warfarin; breakthrough bleeding with oral contraceptives
				
				Food: Enhanced absorption if given with high fat diet
					* Obtain positive identification of organism prior to starting treatment with this drug.
					* Obtain CBC, renal and hepatic tests prior to long-term therapy.
					* Give with food to decrease GI distress.
					* Increase absorption by giving with high-fat meal.
					* Monitor for headache.
					* Observe for side effects.
					* Continue treatment until 2-3 negative weekly cultures and replacement of infected skin, hair, and/or nails.
					* Patient/parent education:
					  - Therapy requires close monitoring by MD.
					  - Therapy lasts between 4 weeks and several months.
					  - Avoid exposure to sun.

Name	Uses	Route and Dose	Adverse Reactions/ Side Effects	Drug or Food Interactions	Nursing Considerations
Generic: Miconazole **Trade:** Monistat Micatin	Antifungal	**IV:** > 1 yr.: 15-40 mg/kg/day equally divided q 8h (max. dose = 15 mg/kg/dose) **Topical:** Apply BID x 2-4 weeks **Intrathecal:** 20 mg/dose q 1-2 days **Vaginal:** 1 applicatorful q HS x 7 days	**CNS:** Dizziness, drowsiness, headache, IT administration - arachnoiditis, transient saddle numbness, 12th cranial nerve palsy, mild third ventricular hemorrhage **GI:** Nausea, vomiting, anorexia **Skin:** Pruritus (IV), irritation, burning, maceration (topical) **Hemic:** Transient decrease in hematocrit, normocytic or microcytic anemia, thrombocytopenia **Other:** Fever, chills, flushing, hyperlipidemia, serum triglycerides, hyponatremia **Local:** Phlebitis	**Drugs:** Altered metabolism if given with cyclosporine, phenytoin, rifampin; antagonized if used with amphotericin B; enhanced anticoagulant effects if used with coumarin drugs. **Foods:** None	* Obtain positive identification of organism prior to starting treatment with this drug. * Obtain baseline hct, hgb, serum electrolytes, and lipids. * Discard IV solution if dark in color. * Infuse over 60 minutes. * Do not mix with other drugs. * Do not use vaginal suppositories with latex diaphragms or condoms. * Monitor for cardiac arrhythmias during infusion. * Monitor for phlebitis. * Observe for side effects. * Monitor hct, hgb, serum electrolytes, and lipids. * Patient/parent education: - Teach proper application of topical forms. - Therapy usually lasts between 6 and 12 weeks. - If no improvement in 2 weeks, contact MD. - Wear panty liner to prevent staining of underwear. - Do not apply other OTC topical medications without consulting MD.

Name	Uses	Route and Dose	Adverse Reactions/ Side Effects	Drug or Food Interactions	Nursing Considerations
Generic: Nystatin Trade: Mycostatin	Antifungal	PO: Premature infants, neonates: 100,000 U QID Infants: 200,000 units QID Children & Adults: 500,000 units QID Topical: Apply sufficient amount to cover affected area QD Vaginal: 1 suppository or applicatorful q HS x 7 days	GI: Transient nausea, vomiting, diarrhea Skin: Rare topical irritation usually a reaction to preservatives	Drugs: None noted. Foods: None	* Obtain positive identification of organism but may start therapy prior to identification. * Assist patient in having good oral hygiene. * Do not give fluids for 30 minutes following administration. * If child is old enough, have him swish medication in for as long as possible before swallowing. * Provide good oral hygiene 30 mins following administration (many solutions contain up to 50% sucrose). * Wear gloves when applying topically. * If using powder, do not inhale particles. * Do not cover areas with occlusive dressings. * Give vaginal medication during menstruation. * If skin irritation occurs, discontinue and notify MD. * Patient/parent education: - Teach proper application of topical forms. - Continue medication for full course of therapy as prescribed by MD. - Teach good oral hygiene to prevent reinfection. - Wear panty liner to prevent staining of underwear. - Do not apply other OTC topical medications without consulting MD. - Discard or disinfect toothbrush. - Children should not share towels or clothes during treatment.

Table 4. ANTIVIRALS

Name	Uses	Route and Dose	Adverse Reactions/ Side Effects	Drug or Food Interactions	Nursing Considerations

Generic: Ribavirin
 	
Trade: Virazole
	Antiviral used to treat severe lower respiratory infections caused by respiratory syncytial virus (RSV).	**Inhalation:** 190 mcg/L in mist by Viratek small-particle aerosol generator (SPAG-2) per oxygen hood or face mask at a rate of 12.5 - L mist per minute over 12-18 h for a minimum of 3 days and a maximum of 7 days.	**CV:** Hypotension, <u>cardiac arrest</u>
			Resp: Worsening of respiratory function, dyspnea, <u>bacterial pneumonia, pneumothorax,</u> ventilator dependence
			Skin: Rash
			Hemic: Reticulocytosis, anemia
			Sensory: Erythema of eyelids, conjunctivitis
				Drugs: Studies are incomplete although it appears that the antiviral activity of zidovudine against HIV may be antagonized and the antiviral activity of other agents may be enhanced.
				
				Foods: None
					* Treatment may be started prior to obtaining culture but should not continue for more than 24 hrs before positive confirmation of RSV infection.
					* Do not use with mild or moderate infections.
					* Most effective in the first 3 days of infection.
					* Drug is teratogenic in animal studies; question family and visitors about possible pregnancy.
					* Pregnant staff members should not have prolonged contact with mist.
					* Staff should not wear soft contact lens while caring for child (causes crystallization of contacts).
					* Do not administer with any other aerosol medications.
					* Assess respiratory function carefully.
					* Informed consent is required by the FDA prior to administering to any child on a ventilator.
					* Patient/parent education:
					  - Give information about disease process.
					  - Provide information on isolation procedures.
					  - Provide information about drug therapy.

Name	Uses	Route and Dose	Adverse Reactions/ Side Effects	Drug or Food Interactions	Nursing Considerations

Generic: Acyclovir
 	
Trade: Zorivax
	Antiviral used to treat cytomegalovirus and herpes simplex infections and varicella zoster infections in immunocompromised children.	**PO:**
		Genital HSV:
		200 mg x 5 doses/day for 5 days
		
		IV:
		Neonates: 30 mg/kg/day equally divided q 8h
		Children < 12 years: 750 mg/m²/day equally divided q 8h
		Children > 5 years: 5 mg/kg equally divided q 8h
		
		IV:
		Neonates: 30 mg/kg/24 hrs divided every 8 hrs for 14-21 days
		Children: Mucocutaneous: 15 mg/kg/24 hrs divided every 8 hrs for 5-10 days
		Encephalitis: 30 mg/kg/24 hrs divided every 8 hrs for 14-21 days
		
		Oral:
		Genital HSV: 25-80 mg/kg/ 24 hrs divided every 8 hrs for 7-10 days
			CNS: Headache, dizziness, fatigue, insomnia, irritability, depression, IV administration - lethargy, obtundation, tremors, confusion, hallucinations, agitation, seizures, coma
			CV: Hypotension, palpitations
			GI: Nausea, vomiting, diarrhea
			Hepatic: Transient rise in SGOT, SGPT, alkaline phosphatase
			GU: Hematuria, transient rise in serum creatinine
			Skin: Rash, urticaria, acne, accelerated hair loss
			Hemic: Thrombocytosis, thrombocytopenia, leukopenia, lymphopenia
			Musculoskeletal: Arthralgia, pars planitis, muscle cramps, leg pain
			Other: Fever, sore throat, lymphadenopathy, superficial thrombophlebitis
				Drugs: Half-life and renal clearance increased if given with probenecid; use cautiously with children who have had previous interferon or cytotoxic induced neurologic reactions; cautious use in children receiving intrathecal methotrexate.
				
				Foods: None
					* Record appearance and number of lesions.
					* Confirm diagnosis with culture of lesions.
					* Give drug at first sign of infection (tingling, burning, itching, or pain).
					* Do not give drug SC, IM, ID, or ophthalmically.
					* Do not give IV push; administer over 1 hr.
					* Wear gloves when applying topical drug (HS virus has been reported to have survived 88 hrs on inanimate objects).
					* Provide adequate hydration during and after IV administration.
					* Monitor for CNS symptoms.
					* Assess urinary function (I&O, renal function studies).
					* Avoid extravasation.
					* Patient/parent education:
					  - Provide information on application of drug to avoid spread of disease.
					  - Teach good handwashing technique.
					  - Children should have separate wash cloths and towels and should not share clothing.
					  - Provide information/education on how the disease is spread, S&S of infection, prevention of transmission to others.

Table 5. CNS MEDICATIONS

Name	Uses	Route and Dose	Adverse Reactions/ Side Effects	Drug or Food Interactions	Nursing Considerations
Generic: Caffeine **Trade:** Caffedrine	CNS stimulant used to treat neonatal apnea.	Oral, IV: Loading Dose: 10-20 mg/kg as caffeine citrate or (5-10 mg/kg) as caffeine base. Maintenance Dose: 5-10 mg/kg as caffeine citrate daily or 2.5-5 mg/kg as caffeine base every day starting 24 hrs after the loading dose.	**CNS:** Insomnia, restlessness, nervousness, delirium, dizziness, tremors, headache, confusion, irritability, seizures, anxiety, tinnitus **CV:** Increased pulse, arrhythmia **GI:** Abdominal distention and vomiting in neonates, nausea, diarrhea, gastric irritation **GU:** Bacteriuria, nephritis, frequency **Other:** Kernicterus in neonates	**Drugs:** Increased inotropic effects of beta blockers; increased metabolism of barbiturates; increased side effects of other xanthines (i.e., aminophylline); inhibits calcium absorption; increased half-life if given with disulfiram. **Foods:** None	* Take baseline vital signs. * Do not use during respiratory and cardiac failure. * Use only citrated injection for neo-natal apnea (other preparations may cause kernicterus). * Give slowly. * Monitor vital signs during administration. * Draw blood levels 24 hrs following initial dose and then 1-2x week.

Name	Uses	Dose and Route	Adverse Reactions/ Side Effects	Drug or Food Interactions	Nursing Considerations
Generic: Carbamazinepine Trade: Tegretol	Anticonvulsant used to treat psychomotor, clonic-tonic, and mixed seizures. Also provides pain relief from trigeminal neuralgia. Also used without FDA approval to treat pain and symptoms of multiple sclerosis, hemifacial spasm, dystonia, and antidiuretic effects in diabetes insipidus.	PO: < 6 yrs: 5 mg/kg/day increasing to 10 mg/kg/day in 5-7 days prn and then to 20 mg/kg/day in 5-7 days prn. 6-12 yrs: 100 mg BID increasing by 100 mg/day in weekly intervals prn. Doses should not > 1 g/day and should be given TID or QID if daily dose >200 mg. Usual maintenance dose is 400-800 mg/day. > 12 yrs: 200 mg BID increasing by up to 200 mg/day prn in weekly intervals. Doses should not > 1 g/day for patients 13-15 yrs and 1.2 g/day for > 15 yrs. Doses should be given TID or QID if daily dose > 400 mg. Usual maintenance dose is 800-1200 mg/day.	CNS: Ataxia and dizziness (plasma levels ≤ 10 mg/ml), nystagmus (plasma levels 4 mg/ml), drowsiness, vertigo, diplopia, speech changes, involuntary movements; behavior changes, weakness, headache, depression, trembling, hallucinations CV: CHF, hypertension, hypotension, thrombophlebitis, arrhythmia, chest pain, changes in heart rate GI: Nausea, vomiting, diarrhea, GI pain, constipation, dry mouth, sore throat, mouth ulcers Resp: Dyspnea, pneumonia Hepatic: Jaundice, hepatitis, abnormal liver function tests GU: Frequency, retention, oliguria, renal failure, SIADH Skin: Rash, urticaria, pigmentation changes (especially with light exposure), alopecia, worsening of lupus erythematosus Hemic: Aplastic anemia, leukopenia, eosinophilia, thrombocytopenia, agranulocytosis, leukocytosis Other: Fever, aching joints, muscle cramps, ocular changes	Drugs: Decreased serum concentrations if used with phenytoin, phenobarbital, doxycycline, and warfarin; breakthrough bleeding with oral contraceptives; increased serum levels when used with verapamil or erythromycin; do not give with monoamine oxidase inhibitors. Foods: None	* Take baseline CBC, platelet, reticulocyte, iron studies, liver function tests, BUN, ECG, UA, EEG, and eye studies. * This medication is used only with children who have had serious side effects or no change in seizure activity when utilizing other anticonvulsant medications. * Should not be used in children suffering from mixed seizure disorders as it worsens seizure activity. * Give with food to increase absorption. * Monitor CBC, platelets, reticulocytes, and iron counts q week x 3 months and then monthly. Drug should be dc'd if RBC is < 4 million/mm³, hct < 32%, hgb < 11 g/dl, WBC < 4000/mm³, reticulocyte < 20,000/mm³, platelet count < 100,000/mm³, or serum iron is > 150 mg/dl. * Regularly monitor liver function tests, renal studies (including BUN and UA), serum electrolytes, and eye studies. * Patient/parent education: - Take drug only as directed. - Do not operate machinery or drive a car. - Do not stop medication suddenly. - Avoid sunlight exposure. - Notify MD immediately if bleeding, bruising, fever, sore throat or fatigue occur. - See MD regularly. - Wear bracelet stating that patient suffers from seizures and takes anticonvulsant medication.

Name	Uses	Route and Dose	Adverse Reactions/ Side Effects	Drug or Food Interactions	Nursing Considerations
Generic: Clonazepan **Trade:** Clonapin	Anticonvulsant used in absence, akinetic, and myoclonic seizures. Also used without FDA approval to treat tonic-clonic, psychomotor, and infantile spasm seizures.	**PO:** **< 10 yrs or 30 kg:** 0.01 - 0.03 mg/kg/day initially in 2-3 doses (not to exceed 0.05 mg/kg/day in 2-3 doses); dosage is increased no more than 0.5 mg q 3 days and maintenance dose should not exceed 0.2 mg/kg/day **Older children:** 1.5 mg/day initially with dosage increased 0.5-0.0 mg q 3 days and maintenance should not exceed 20 mg/day.	**CNS:** Sedation, drowsiness, ataxia, behavior changes especially in those with brain damage, mental retardation, or mental illness, aggression, irritability, hyperactivity, confusion, depression, headache, dizziness, tremor, vertigo, insomnia **CV:** Palpitation **GI:** Constipation, gastritis, anorexia, nausea, dry mouth, thirst, sore gums **Resp:** Increased secretions, dyspnea, difficulty swallowing **Hepatic:** Hepatomegaly, liver enzyme changes **GU:** Dysuria, enuresis, retention, nocturia **Skin:** Hirsutism or hair loss, rash **Hemic:** Anemia, leukopenia, thrombocytopenia, eosinophilia **Other:** Fever, dehydration, lymphadenopathy	**Drugs:** Increased depressant effects if used with CNS depressants; increases serum phenytoin levels; increased serum levels when used with cimetidine or disulfiram; decreased serum levels of both if used with carbamazepine. **Foods:** None	* Take baseline weight, height, liver function studies, and CBC. * Record seizure activity. * Tolerance may develop as soon as 3 months, necessitating changes in drug regime. * Measure height and weight regularly. * Monitor liver function studies and CBC periodically. * Monitor behavior changes. * Patient/parent education: - Take drug only as directed. - Do not operate machinery or drive a car. - Do not stop medication suddenly. - Report continuing symptoms of drowsiness and ataxia (these should decrease as therapy continues). - Avoid alcohol, CNS depressants, and other medications unless prescribed by MD. - Wear bracelet stating that patient suffers from seizures and takes anticonvulsant medication.

Name	Uses	Dose and Route	Adverse Reactions/ Side Effects	Drug or Food Interactions	Nursing Considerations

Generic: Pentobarbital
 	
Trade: Nembutal
	Short-term treatment of insomnia; preoperative sedation; high dose barbiturate coma for treatment of increased intracranial pressure or status epilepticus unresponsive to other therapy.	Increased intracranial pressure: IV: Initial: 3-5 mg/kg as a single dose; maintenance: 2-3.5 mg/kg/ dose every hour as needed to maintain level between 25 and 40 mcg/ml.
		
		Children: Hypnotic <4 yrs: IM: 2-6 mg/kg/dose divided in 3 doses, up to a max of 100 mg/dose Rectal: 3-6 mg/kg/dose >4 yrs: IM: 2-6 mg/kg/dose, up to a max of 100 mg/dose Rectal: 1.5-3 mg/kg/dose
		
		Adolescents >12 yrs: Conscious sedation: IV: 100 mg prior to a procedure
		
		Preoperative sedation: IM: 150-200 mg
			CNS: Drowsiness, lethargy, headache, vertigo, mental depression, impaired motor skills **CV:** Vasodilation, hypotension **GI:** Nausea, vomiting, diarrhea, constipation **Resp:** Respiratory depression, apnea, bronchospasm, laryngospasm, especially with rapid IV infusion **Hepatic:** Hepatitis, jaundice **Skin:** Thrombophlebitis at IV site, hypersensitivity reaction with skin rash, urticaria, dermatitis, systemic lupus erythematosus	**Drugs:** Potentiates other CNS depressants; decreased GI absorption of dicumarol; decreased levels of corticosteroids; decreased levels of griseofulvin; decreased half-life of doxycycline; decreased effectiveness of birth control pills; increased respiratory depressant effects with other drugs having this effect.
				
				Food: None
					* Take baseline vital signs and assess for allergy to barbiturates and respiratory disease.
					* Take po medications on empty stomach.
					* Check injectable preparations for precipitate.
					* Incompatible with many drugs — do not mix when giving IV.
					* Take vital signs frequently during administration; pulse oximeter.
					* Do not use for longer than 2 weeks to treat insomnia.
					* Monitor for bruising, fever, sore throat, bleeding and discontinue drug if these are present.
					* Observe for skin reactions. These are potentially fatal and drug should be discontinued if they are noted.
					* Patient/parent education:
					  - Take drug only as directed.
					  - Do not operate machinery or drive a car.
					  - Report signs of fever, sore throat, bleeding, bruising, or skin reaction.
					  - Avoid alcohol, CNS depressants, and other medications unless prescribed by MD.
					  - Drug may be habit forming and long-term use requires a slow withdrawal.
					* Avoid rapid IV administration >50 mg/min; intermittent infusion: over 10-30 mins, not to exceed 50 mg/ min; max concentration 50 mg/ml.
					* Suppositories should not be cut.

Name	Uses	Dose and Route	Adverse Reactions/ Side Effects	Drug or Food Interactions	Nursing Considerations
Generic: Phenobarbital **Trade:** Luminal	Management of grand mal, partial seizures and febrile seizures in children; also used as a preoperative sedative and other situations when sedation is needed; a hypnotic; may also be used for prevention and treatment of neonatal hyper-bilirubinemia and lowering of bilrubin in chronic cholestasis.	**Anticonvulsant:** Neonates: Initial 15-20 mg/kg; maintenance: 3-5 mg/kg/24 hrs Infants: 5-8 mg/kg/24 hrs divided 1-2 times/day **Status Epilepticus:** Infants and children: Give 10-20 mg/kg as the initial dose, followed by 5-10 mg/kg/dose at intervals of 20 mins, until seizure controlled or a total dose of 40 mg/kg. **Children:** Sedation: Oral, IM: 2 mg/kg 3 times/day Hypnotic: Oral, IM, IV, SC: 3-5 mg/kg at bedtime Hyperbilirubinemia: Oral, up to 12 yrs: 3-12 mg/kg/day in 2-3 divided doses Preoperative sedation: Oral, IM, IV: 1-3 mg/kg 1-1 1/2 hrs before procedure Anticonvulsant: 3-5 mg/kg/24 hrs divided 1-2 times/day	**CNS:** Drowsiness, ataxia, irritability, headache, paradoxical excitement, hyperactivity, sleep disturbance, impaired memory, school difficulties **GI:** Nausea, vomiting **Hepatic:** Hepatitis, jaundice **GU:** Renal damage **Skin:** Rash, dermatitis **Hemic:** Lowered RBC levels, bone marrow suppression **Metabolic:** Hypocalcemia	**Drugs:** Possibly increases or decreases phenytoin levels; decreases serum levels of corticosteroids, tricyclic antidepressants, griseofulvin, doxycycline, and digoxin; increases depressant effects of alcohol and other CNS depressants. **Food:** None	* Take baseline CBC, liver function tests, UA. * Assess history of child's school performance. * May mix po forms with food. * Inject IM doses deep into large muscle — inadvertent SC injection may cause tissue necrosis. * May mix with most IV solutions. * Use reconstituted solution within 30 minutes and do not use if precipitate noted. * Incompatible with many drugs — do not mix for administration. * IV administration not to exceed 2 mg/kg/min or 30 mg/min. * Monitor level of consciousness. * Monitor vital signs, CBC, liver and renal function tests if on long-term therapy. * Monitor school performance if on long-term therapy. * Observe for signs of hypocalcemia. * Patient/parent education: - Take drug only as directed. - Do not d/c medication, alter dose or change forms without con-sulting MD. - Do not take other drugs or alcohol with this medication. - Report increasing dizziness, lethargy, ataxia, changes in school performance to MD.

Name	Uses	Dose and Route	Adverse Reactions/ Side Effects	Drug or Food Interactions	Nursing Considerations

Generic: Phenytoin
 	
Trade: Dilantin
	Anticonvulsant used for tonic-clonic and partial seizures as well as seizures with nonepilepsy cause.	Status Epilepticus: IV:
		Neonates: Loading dose: 15-20 mg/kg in a single divided dose
		Maintenance, anticonvulsant: 5-8 mg/kg/day in a single dose or divided dose; maintenance, anticonvulsant: 4-7 mg/kg/day in 1-2 divided doses.
		
		Anticonvulsant: Oral:
		Loading dose: 15-20 mg/kg; based on phenytoin serum concentrations and if no doses had been administered in the previous 24 hrs.
		Neonates: Maintenance dose: 5 mg/kg/day in divided doses every 12 hrs.
		Infants >10 days to 3 yrs: Maintenance dose: 8-10 mg/kg/day in divided doses every 8-12 hrs
		Children and Adults: Maintenance dose: 5-8 mg/kg/day in divided doses every 12-24 hrs.
			CNS: Confusion, drowsiness during early therapy, dizziness, headache; nystagmus, diplopia and ataxia indicate intoxication
			CV: Cardiovascular arrest, hypotension with IV use
			GI: Nausea, vomiting, anorexia, decreased sense of taste, weight loss
			Skin: Pain and necrosis at injection site, rash or severe dermatitis with fever, lupus erythematosus, Stevens-Johnson syndrome, hirsutism (particularly in females)
			Hemic: Thrombocytopenia, leukopenia, granulocytopenia, pancytopenia, anemia
			Endocrine: Hyperglycemia
			Other: Lymphadenopathy, hypertrichosis, osteomalacia, gingival hyperplasia
				Drugs: Serum levels decreased by CNS depressants, antacids, barbiturates, folic acid, rifampin, valproic acid (may also increase levels); increased sedation with primidone; may decrease serum digoxin levels; increased levels with disulfiram.
				
				Foods: May interfere with Vitamin D absorption and folic acid metabolism.
					* Take baseline CBC, liver function tests, UA.
					* Assess vital signs before starting IV.
					* Assess previous skin reactions to phenytoin administration.
					* Note type of phenytoin used — chewable tabs and suspension are phenytoin sodium and contain less phenytoin. Bioavailability depends on brand of phenytoin used.
					* PO forms should be given with food to decrease gastric distress.
					* IV solution should be clear or slightly yellow — do not use if any precipitate noted.
					* Give IV no faster than 0.5-1.5 mg/kg/min.
					* Do not mix with other medications.
					* Clear line with normal saline flush before and after IV injection.
					* Monitor CBC, liver functions, and UA if on long-term therapy.
					* Monitor serum drug levels.
					* Patient/parent education:
					  - Take drug only as directed.
					  - Do not d/c medication, alter dose or change forms or brands without consulting MD.
					  - Do not take other drugs or alcohol.
					  " Teach family emergency care for seizures and to report all seizure activity.
					  " Drug can alter alertness — avoid driving and alter activities accordingly.
					  " Teach oral hygiene as soon as teeth erupt.
					  - Report classroom performance.

Name	Uses	Dose and Route	Adverse Reactions/ Side Effects	Drug or Food Interactions	Nursing Considerations

Generic: Valproic acid
 	
Trade: Depakene, Depakote
	Used alone or combined with other CNS medications for simple and complex absence (petit mal) seizures. Also used without FDA approval for other types of seizures.	**PO:** 15 mg/kg/day initially. May be increased by 5-10 mg/kg/day PRN. Should not exceed 60 mg/kg/day. Usually given in 2 divided doses.	**CNS:** Drowsiness, headache, tremor, anxiety, confusion, paresthesia, dizziness, incoordination; hyperactivity and behavior changes more common in children
			GI: Nausea, vomiting, indigestion (common); hypersalivation, anorexia, weight loss, diarrhea, constipation, cramps
			Hepatic: Hepatotoxicity with increased liver enzymes, most common in children < 2 yrs who are receiving other drugs, have metabolic disease or mental retardation
			GU: Enuresis
			Skin: Rash, hair loss or changes, facial swelling
			Hemic: Decreased platelet aggregation and prolonged bleeding time; bruising, thrombocytopenia, leukopenia, eosinophilia, anemia, decreased fibrinogen
				Drugs: Increased CNS depression if used with other CNS depressants; increases phenobarbital and primidone levels; not recommended with clonazepam due to possible seizure activity; may alter binding and action of phenytoin; potentiates MAO inhibitors and antidepressants; use cautiously with anticoagulants; may increase folic acid needs; increased risk of hepatotoxicity in young children taking other anticonvulsants or hepatotoxic medications.
				
				Foods: None
					* Obtain baseline renal and liver function tests, CBC, coagulation tests, and serum ammonia.
					* Do not give medication if abnormal liver function or coagulation tests or hyperammonia.
					* Monitor liver function tests frequently—especially in first 6 months when risk of hepatotoxicity is greatest.
					* Coagulation studies should be monitored periodically and prior to any surgical procedures.
					* Give with food to decrease gastric distress.
					* Patient/parent education:
					  - Take drug only as directed.
					  - Do not change dosage of medication.
					  - Return for scheduled follow up visits.
					  - Avoid OTC medications and alcohol.
					  - Avoid driving and adjust activities due to altered mental alertness.
					  - Notify MD's of use of this medication prior to having surgery or dental work.
					  - Child should wear identification bracelet stating history of seizure activity and use of valproic acid.

Table 6. BRONCHODILATORS/PULMONARY MEDICATIONS

Name	Uses	Route and Dose	Adverse Reactions/ Side Effects	Drug or Food Interactions	Nursing Considerations
Generic:: Acetylcysteine **Trade:** Mucomyst	Mucolytic used to decrease the viscosity of respiratory secretions. Used in treatment of cystic fibrosis, bronchitis, pneumonia, tuberculosis, mucous obstruction atelectasis, and emphysema. Also used to prevent hepatotoxicity in treatment of acetaminophen overdose.	**PO:** **Acetaminophen Overdose:** 140 mg/kg initially followed by 70 mg/kg q 4 hrs x 17 doses **Inhalation:** **Nebulized solution:** 3-5 mg of 20% solution or 6-10 mg 10% solution TID or QID **Tent or Croupette:** 300 ml of 10 or 20% solution **Intratracheal:** 1-2 ml of 10 or 20% solution q 1-4h	**CNS:** Drowsiness **GI:** Nausea, vomiting, stomatitis **Resp:** Rhinorrhea, bronchospasm (more common in asthmatics), hemoptysis **Skin:** Urticaria (generalized) **Other:** Fever, chills	**Drugs:** Decreased effectiveness if used with activated charcoal; incompatible with amphotericin B, chlortetracycline HCl, erythromycin lactobionate, oxytetracycline HCl, ampicillin, tetracycline, iodized oil, trypsin, and hydrogen peroxide. **Foods:** None	* Assess baseline respiratory rate and characteristics. * Assess cough for frequency and type and amount and type of secretions. * Draw serum drug levels if acetaminophen ingestion. Treatment may start prior to receiving lab results. Do not delay if ingestion within 24 hours. * Drug most effective if given within 10-12 hours of reported ingestion. May dilute solution for overdose treatment with soft drinks or juice. Use within 1 hour of dilution. * Drug has foul odor (rotten eggs) so administer in container with lid and straw. * If dose vomited within 1 hour, repeat. * If used for overdosage, monitor for other signs of acetaminophen toxicity. * If given via NG or OG tube, dilute prior to administration to prevent irritation or sclerosing of duodenum. * Do not administer via hand held nebulizer due to large particle size. * Use only plastic or glass nebulizer * Do not use heated nebulizer. * Administer with compressed air or oxygen. Administer with caution in patients with CO_2 retention. * Have patient clear airway prior to administration. * Keep continuous nebulizer full to prevent impedance of drug delivery. * Patient/parent education: - Follow teaching plan. - Have regular medical follow up.

Name	Uses	Route and Dose	Adverse Reactions/ Side Effects	Drug or Food Interactions	Nursing Considerations
Generic: Aminophylline Trade: Aminophyllin, Somophyllin-DF	Bronchodilator used in treatment of bronchial asthma, chronic bronchitis, and emphysema. Used for apnea of prematurity and bradycardia in neonates.	PO: 1-9 yrs: 20 mg/kg/day q 6h 9-16 yrs: 16 mg/kg/day q 6h > 16 years (adult): 12 mg/kg/day q 6h IV: * Neonatal apnea: loading dose = 4-6 mg/kg x 1 dose (each 1 mg/kg will raise serum dr level 2 mcg/ml) Maintenance: Preterm infants to 40 weeks postnatal age: 1 mg/kg q 12h Term newborns to 4 weeks postnatal age: 1-2 mg/kg q 8h 4-8 weeks postnatal age: 1-3 mg/kg q 8h * Bronchospasm: loading dose = 6 mg/kg x 1 dose Maintenance: Neonates up to 24 days: 1.25 mg/kg q 12h Neonates > 24 days: 1.9 mg/kg q 12h 1-9 yrs: 1 mg/kg/hr 9-12 yrs: 0.9 mg/kg/hr 12-16 yrs (nonsmoker): 0.6 mg/kg/hr 12-16 yrs (smoker): 0.9 mg/kg/hr * Doses must be individualized and based on serum drug levels	CNS: Headaches, restlessness, dizziness, irritability, insomnia, muscle twitching, seizures CV: Palpitations, sinus tachycardia, extrasystoles, flushing, marked hypotension, circulatory failure, cardiac arrest GI: Nausea, vomiting, bitter aftertaste, epigastric pain, anorexia, diarrhea Resp: Tachypnea GU: Albuminuria Skin: Urticaria, exfoliative dermatitis Other: Hyperglycemia, SIADH, local redness and pain at IV site	Drugs: Serum drug levels increased by phenytoin and barbiturates; decreases effectiveness of lithium and furosemide; beta-adrenergic blockers (especially propranolol and nadolol) may induce bronchospasms when used concurrently; decreased hepatic clearance with erythromycin, cimetidine, troleandomycin; enhances toxic potential of cardiac glycosides; increased CNS stimulation with adrenergics. Food: None	* Assess respiratory status and vital signs. * Weigh patient. * If child is currently taking theophylline, determine when amount and time last dose given. * Withhold dose from neonates with heart rate > 180. * Delayed absorption if given with food, but may administer with meals if GI irritation present. * If IV, do not administer faster than 25 mg/minute. * IV administration rate usually 25-30 minutes. * Continuous IV infusion usually given at rate of 0.9-1.5 mg/kg/hour. * Do not use continuous infusion for neonates. * Monitor respiratory status. * Monitor serum drug levels frequently and maintain between 10-20 mcg/ml. * Check with pharmacist prior to mixing with any drug. * Patient/parent education: - Report any CNS, cardiac, or GI side effects to MD. - Monitor respiratory response. - Maintain hydration and weight. - Do not use any OTC drugs containing ephedrine. - Take as directed and at same time each day to maintain levels.

Name	Uses	Route and Dose	Adverse Reactions/ Side Effects	Drugs or Food Interactions	Nursing Considerations
Generic: Epinephrine **Trade:** Adrenalin, EpiPen Jr.; Vaponefrin	Bronchospasms, anaphylactic reactions, cardiac arrest, refractory shock, hypotension, management of open angle (chronic simple) glaucoma.	Neonates: IV or intrathecal: 0.01-0.03 mg/kg (1:10,000 solution) every 3-5 mins as needed; dilute intrathecal doses to 1-2 mL of normal saline. Infants & children: Bronchodilator: SC: 10 mcg/kg, single doses not to exceed 0.5 mg Bradycardia: IV: 0.01 mg/kg of 1:10,000 solution; max: 1 mg. Intrathecal: 0.1 mg/kg of 1:10,000 solution; doses as high as 0.2 mg/kg may be effective. Asystole or pulselessness: IV or intraosseous: First dose: 0.01 mg/kg (1:10,000 solution); subsequent doses: 0.1 mg/kg (1:10,000 solution); doses as high as 0.2 mg/kg may be effective, repeat every 3-5 mins as needed. Intrathecal: 0.1 mg/kg (1:10,000 solution); doses as high as 0.2 mg/kg may be effective. Inhalation (racemic epinephrine): <2 yrs: 0.25 mL in 3mL normal saline; each treatment is ordered individually. >2 yrs and adolescents: 0.5 mL in 3 mL normal saline; each treatment is ordered individually.	**CNS:** Anxiety, restlessness, dizziness, headache, excitability, weakness, syncope, convulsions, fever, chills **CV:** Tachycardia, palpitations, increased blood pressure, flushing, EKG changes, chest pain, irregular pulse **Resp:** Dyspnea, rebound bronchospasm after withdrawal of inhalation therapy **GI:** Nausea, vomiting **Skin:** Necrosis at injection site with repeated injections; pale cold skin **Sensory:** Blurred vision, enlarged pupils **Other:** Prolonged use can lead to metabolic acidosis	**Drugs:** Additive effects with other sympatho-mimetics; decreased respiratory and cardiac effects with beta adrenergic blockers; severe hypoten-sion and tachycardia if given with rapid-acting vasodilators; decreased effects with antihyper-tensives; increased cardiac effects observed if given with some general anesthetics; increased cardiac effects with cardiac glycosides, tricyclic antidepressants, antihista-mines, and thyroid medica-tions; monitor EKG if given with digitalis; added CNS effects with other CNS stimulants and xanthines; increased insulin needs with diabetes. **Foods:** None	* Baseline vital signs, especially pulse and B/P. * Evaluate and monitor EKG, blood gases, CVP, and urine output. * Monitor blood glucose in diabetic patients closely. * Patient/parent education: - Teach correct inhalation technique. - Do not use solutions that are dis-colored or have precipitate. - Seek medical attention if asthma not improved in 20 minutes following administration. - Do not exceed recommended dose. - Rinse mouth with water following each dose to prevent dryness.

Name	Uses	Route and Dose	Adverse Reactions/ Side Effects	Drug or Food Interactions	Nursing Considerations
Generic: Metaproterenol **Trade:** Alupent	Bronchodilator used to manage asthma; prevention of exercise induced asthma, and to enhance therapeutic effects of theophylline	**PO:** < 6 yrs: 1.3 - 2.6 mg/kg/day 6-9 yrs (27.3 kg): 10 mg 3-4 times/day > 9 yrs: 20 mg 3-4 times/day **Inhalation:** 12 yrs **Aerosol:** 2-3 inhalations q 3-4h (max. dose 12 inhalations/day) **Nebulizer solution:** 0.2-0.3 ml of 5% solution in 2.5 ml of NS or 2.5 ml of 0.6% solution q 4-6h	**CNS:** Nervousness, tremors, dizziness, headache, drowsiness **CV:** Tachycardia, palpitations, hypertension, cardiac arrest (overdosage) **GI:** Nausea, vomiting, bad taste **Other:** Muscle cramps	**Drugs:** Additive effects if used with other sympathomimetic amines; bronchodilation effects antagonized by effects of beta adrenergic blocking agents **Foods:** None	* Assess respiratory status. * Obtain baseline heart rate. * Do not crush PO tabs. May be administered with food. * Side effects more common with oral forms. * Shake inhalation forms well prior to administration. * Monitor respiratory response. * Maintain hydration. * May use PO and inhalation forms concurrently. * Patient/parent education: - Teach correct inhalation technique. - Do not exceed recommended dose. - Discontinue if paradoxical bronchospasms noted. - Do not use this with any other inhalers.

Name	Uses	Route and Dose	Adverse Reactions/ Side Effects	Drug or Food Interactions	Nursing Considerations

Generic: Terbutaline sulfate
 	
Trade: Brethine, Brethaire
	Bronchial dilator used to treat asthma and emphysema.	**PO:**
		> 12 yrs: 0.05 mg/kg/dose TID (max. dose — 7.5 mg/day)
		
		SC:
		< 12 yrs: 0.005-0.010 mg/kg/dose (max. dose 0.25 mg/dose q 15-20 minutes BID)
		> 12 yrs: 3.5-5 mcg/kg (max. dose 0.5 mg in 4h)
		
		Inhalation:
		2 inhalations (400 mcg) q 4-6h
			CNS: Nervousness, tremors, dizziness, headache, lethargy, sweating.
			CV: Palpitations, <u>tachycardia</u>, <u>dysrhythmia</u>
			GI: Nausea, vomiting
			Sensory: Dry nose, mouth and throat; tinnitus
				Drugs: Hypertensive crisis with MAO inhibitors; additive effects with other sympathomimetic amines; antagonized bronchodilator effects with beta adrenergic blocking agents.
				
				Foods: None
					* Assess respiratory status.
					* Obtain baseline heart rate.
					* Do not crush extended-release tabs.
					* May crush other tabs and mix with food.
					* Do not use SC solution if discolored.
					* **SC doses must be checked with an RN prior to administration. Errors in decimal points may be fatal!**
					* Monitor cardiac response with SC route.
					* May repeat SC dose if no improvement in 15-30 minutes.
					* Do not repeat if no improvement after second dose.
					* Maintain hydration.
					* Monitor response.
					* Patient/parent education:
					  - Teach correct inhalation technique.
					  - Do not exceed recommended dose.
					  - Contact MD if symptoms worsen. Discontinue if paradoxical bronchospasms noted.
					  - Do not use this with any other inhalers.

Name	Uses	Route and Dose	Adverse Reactions/ Side Effects	Drug or Food Interactions	Nursing Considerations
Generic: Theophylline **Trade:** Slo-bid Theo-Dur Slo-Phyllin-12	Bronchodilator used to treat bronchial asthma, chronic bronchitis, and emphysema; apnea of prematurity and bradycardia in preterm infants; bronchial spasms in cystic fibrosis.	**PO:** Bronchospasm: Loading dose: 0.8 mg/kg/dose Maintenance: Birth-2 mos: 3-6 mg/kg/day q 8h; 2-6 mo: 6-5 mg/kg/ day q 6h; 6-12 mo: 15-22 mg/kg/day q 6h; 1 - 9 yrs: 20-22 mg/kg/day q 6h (max. dose 24 mg/kg/day); 12-16 yrs: 16-18 mg/kg/day q 6h; > 16 yrs: 13 mg/kg/day q 6h (max. dose 900 mg/day) **Dosing is the same for extended release tabs but they are given q 8-12h** **PO, IV:** Neonatal apnea: Loading dose: 4 mg/kg Maintenance: Preterm infants: 1 mg/kg q 12h; Term infants: 1-2 mg/kg q 8h; 4-8 weeks postnatal: 1-3 mg/kg q 6h **IV:** Bronchospasm: Loading dose: 4.7 mg/kg x 1 dose Maintenance: 6 mo.-9 yrs: 1.2 mg/kg/hr x 12h then 1 mg/kg/hr; 9-16 yrs: 1 mg/ kg/hr x 12h then 0.8 mg/kg/ hr; > 16 yrs (nonsmoker): 0.7 mg/kg/hr x 12h then 0.5 mg/ kg/hr	**CNS:** Headaches, restlessness, dizziness, irritability, insomnia, muscle twitching, <u>seizures</u> **CV:** Palpitations, <u>sinus tachycardia, extrasystoles, flushing, marked hypotension, circulatory failure, cardiac arrest</u> **GI:** Nausea, vomiting, bitter aftertaste, epigastric pain, anorexia, diarrhea **Resp:** Tachypnea **Skin:** Urticaria, exfoliative dermatitis **Other:** Hyperglycemia, SIADH, pain and redness at IV site	**Drugs:** Serum levels decreased by phenytoin and barbiturates; decreases therapeutic effectiveness of lithium and furosemide; may induce bronchospasm when used with beta-adrenergic blockers; decreased hepatic clearance with erythromycin, cimetidine, troleandomycin; increased CNS stimulation with adrenergics; increased metabolism with phenobarbital. **Foods:** Delayed clearance with charcoal-broiled foods.	* Assess respiratory status and vital signs. * Weigh patient. * If child is currently taking theophylline, determine when amount and time last dose given. * Do not allow child to swallow chewable forms whole. * Withhold dose from neonates with heart rate > 180. * Delayed absorption if given with food, but may administer with meals if GI irritation present. * If IV, <u>do not administer faster than 25 mg/minute.</u> * IV administration rate usually 25-30 minutes. * Continuous IV rate = 0.9-1.5 mg/ kg/hr. * Do not use continuous infusion for neonates. * Monitor respiratory status. * Monitor serum drug levels frequently and maintain between 10-20 mcg/ml. * Check with pharmacist prior to mixing with any drug. * Incompatible with acid solutions. * Patient/parent education: - Report any CNS, cardiac, or GI side effects to MD. - Monitor respiratory response. - Maintain hydration and weight. - Do not use any OTC drugs containing ephedrine. - Take as directed and at same time each day to maintain levels.

TABLE 7. CARDIOVASCULAR MEDICATIONS

Name	Uses	Route and Dose	Adverse Reactions/ Side Effects	Drug or Food Interactions	Nursing Considerations
Generic: Atropine Trade: Isopto Atropine	Anticholinergic used to treat vagally induced bradycardia, decrease smooth muscle contractions in GI and GU tracts, decrease secretions in respiratory and GI tracts, and occasionally as a bronchodilator.	**PO:** **Antimuscarinic:** 0.01 mg/kg not to exceed 0.4 mg q 4 -6h **SC:** **Antimuscarinic:** 0.01 mg/kg not to exceed 0.4 mg - may repeat q 4 - 6h **Preop:** < 3kg: 0.1 mg 7 - 9 kg: 0.2 mg 12 - 16 kg: 0.3 mg 20 - 27 kg: 0.4 mg 32 kg: 0.5 mg 41 kg: 0.4 mg **IV:** **Dysrhythmias:** 0.01 - 0.03 mg/kg **Cardiac arrest:** 0.02 mg/kg with a minimum dose of 0.1 mg and maximum dose of 1.0 mg **Inhalation:** 0.05 mg/kg in saline q 6 - 8h	**CNS:** Atropine psychosis, CNS stimulation, restlessness, combativeness, confusion, hallucination, weakness, dizziness, insomnia, headache, paradoxical excitement **CV:** Tachycardia, bradycardia with low doses or slow injection, palpitation **GI:** Nausea, vomiting, loss of taste, bloating, dry mouth, constipation, paralytic ileus **GU:** Urinary retention **Skin:** Hot dry skin, rash, urticaria, dermatitis **Sensory:** Mydriasis, blurred vision, cyclopegia, photophobia, local irritation of eye with topical administration	**Drugs:** Increased effect with MAO inhibitors, increased effects of nitrofurantoin, increased intraocular pressure with other drugs having the same effect, delayed excretion with medications causing urinary alkalinization, decreased absorption with antacids, increased chance of constipation with narcotics. **Foods:** None	* Assess vital signs prior to and frequently following administration. * Give po forms 30 min prior to meals and HS. * Perform good oral hygiene. * Will remain stable for 15 minutes when mixed with other preop medications. * Have patient void before administering preoperatively. * Incompatible with sodium bicarbonate and epinephrine. * Monitor intake and output. * Evaluate bowel sounds and function. * Patient/parent education: - Take only as directed. - Notify MD if side effects occur. - Do not take antacids and antidiarrheals within 1 hour of atropine. - Avoid strenuous activity/exercise. - Avoid hot weather. - Rise to standing position slowly. - Inform of possibility of photophobia. - Avoid operating heavy machinery.

Name	Uses	Route and Dose	Adverse Reactions/ Side Effects	Drug or Food Interactions	Nursing Considerations
Generic: Digoxin **Trade:** Lanoxin, Lanoxicaps, SK-digoxin	Cardiac glycoside used to increase myocardial contractility, increase automaticity, reduce excitability and conduction velocity, and prolong refractory period. Also acts to retain sodium and excrete potassium from myocardium. Used to treat congestive heart failure and to control ventricular rate in atrial flutter and fibrillation.	**PO:** **Digitalizing Dose:** Preterm infants: 20 mcg/kg Neonates: 30 mcg/kg < 2 yrs: 40 - 50 mcg/kg 2 - 10 yrs: 30 - 40 mcg/kg > 10 yrs: 0.75 - 1.25 mg These are administered as 1/2 the total dose initially followed by 1/4 the dose q 8 - 18h x 2 **Maintenance dose:** Preterm infants: 5 mcg/kg/day divided q 12h Neonates: 8 - 10 mcg/kg/day divided q 12h < 2 yrs: 10 - 12 mcg/kg/day divided q 12h 2 - 10 yrs: 8 - 10 mcg/kg/day divided q 12h > 10 yrs: 0.125 -0.25 mg q day **IV,IM:** IV or IM doses are 75% of total PO doses except in the > 10 yr group, when IV,IM = PO	**CNS:** Tiredness, weakness, headache, confusion, depression, fainting, facial neuralgia, paresthesias, hallucinations, agitation **CV:** Bradycardia, dysrhythmias, hypotension, tachycardia **GI:** Nausea, vomiting, anorexia, stomach pain, diarrhea **Sensory:** Blurred vision, halos	**Drugs:** Antacids, kaolin-pectin, cholestyramine, and metroclopramide may decrease absorption of digoxin; quinidine, indomethacin, verapimil, amiodarone, erythromycin, tetracycline, and spironolactone may increase digoxin serum concentration; penicillamine may decrease digoxin's pharmacologic effects. **Foods:** Meals containing increased fiber (bran) or foods high in pectin may decrease oral absorption of digoxin; avoid natural licorice (causes sodium and water retention and increases potassium loss); maintain adequate amounts of potassium in diet to decrease risk of hypokalemia.	* Assess baseline vital signs and ECG. * Obtain baseline serum electrolytes, hepatic and renal function studies. * Hydrate if hypovolemic. * May take with food. * Use calibrated dropper if giving elixir. * Ensure that digoxin not digitoxin tablets are administered. * Dilute IV doses with at least 4x the volume and administer over at least 5 min * Assess apical pulse for one full minute prior to administering digoxin. * Withhold dose if pulse is below normal for age group (often 100 beats/min in children). * Monitor ECG during IV administration. * Monitor serum electrolytes and hepatic and renal functions, particularly if patient taking diuretics. * Monitor serum digoxin levels carefully (levels > 2ng/ml are toxic). * Monitor for tachycardia in young children and stomach upset or bradycardia in older children which may indicate toxicity. * Patient/parent education: - If ordered by MD, teach parents to assess apical pulse for 1 min prior to administering dose; do so at same time each day. - Notify MD and withhold medication if nausea and vomiting occur. - Teach correct measurement and administration. - Teach signs of congestive heart failure. - Due to high risk of accidental poisoning, keep medication out of reach and have syrup of ipecac available. - Wear medical ID bracelet.

Name	Uses	Route and Dose	Side Effects	Interactions	Considerations
Generic: Dobutamine **Trade:** Dobutrex	Catecholamine and cardiac stimulant that increases contractility, stroke volume and cardiac output and decreases peripheral vascular resistance with minimal effects on B/P. Used to treat cardiac failure with resultant low cardiac output.	**IV: Children:** 2.5-15 mcg/kg/min **Neonates:** 3-20 mcg/kg/min. Titrate to desired response.	**CNS:** Headache, paresthesia **CV:** Ectopic beats, tachycardia, angina, palpitations, hypertension **GI:** Nausea **Resp:** Dyspnea	**Drugs:** Decreased effects if used with beta-adrenergic blockers; ventricular dysrhythmias with halothane or cyclopropane anesthesia; increased cardiac output and decreased pulmonary wedge pressure with nitroprusside; increased pressor effects if used with MAO inhibitors and tricyclic antidepressants. **Food:** None	* Monitor vital signs including EKG, cardiac output, skin temperature, peripheral pulses and pulmonary wedge pressure at least q 1 hour. * Patient must be continuously monitored and on a cardiac monitor. * Correct hypovolemia prior to starting medication. * Use prepared solutions within 24 hrs. * Incompatible with many medications—check with pharmacist prior to mixing with other medications or solutions. * Strict intake and output.
Generic: Dopamine **Trade:** Intropin	Precursor to norepinephrine that increases myocardial contractility, stroke volume, and cardiac output by beta adrenergic action. Will increase renal and coronary arterial perfusion at low doses and will cause vasoconstriction at high doses. Used to treat cardiogenic shock and congestive heart failure.	**IV:** Increased renal and coronary artery perfusion: 1-5 mcg/kg/min Increased cardiac output: 5-10 mcg/kg/min Increased peripheral vascular resistance and cardiac output: > 10 mcg/kg/min	**CNS:** Nervousness, headache, numbness or tingling of fingers or toes **CV:** Chest pain, hypotension, irregular pulse, hypertension and tachycardia with rapid infusion, bradycardia, palpitations **Resp:** Dyspnea **GI:** Nausea, vomiting **Skin:** Color changes or pain from vasoconstriction, gangrene in extremities with prolonged use, tissue necrosis with necrosis	**Drugs:** Prolonged effects with MAO inhibitors, decreased cardiac effects if used with beta-adrenergics, hypotension and bradycardia with IV phenytoin, increased chance of dysrhythmias with digitalis and guanethidine, ventricular dysrhythmias and hypertension with halothane or cyclopropane anesthetics, potentiates diuretics and thyroid medications. **Foods:** None	* Monitor vital signs including EKG, cardiac output, skin temperature, peripheral pulses and pulmonary wedge pressure at least q 1 hour. * Patient must be continuously monitored and on a cardiac monitor. * Correct hypovolemia prior to starting medication. * Monitor IV frequently for extravasation. * Monitor carefully for decreased circulation in extremities. * Incompatible with alkaline medications — check with pharmacist prior to mixing with other medications or solutions. * Strict intake and output.

Name	Uses	Route and Dose	Adverse Reactions/ Side Effects	Drug or Food Interactions	Nursing Considerations
Generic: Isoproterenol **Trade:** Isuprel	Beta-adrenergic stimulant used to reduce peripheral vascular resistance and increase the force of cardiac contractions without vasoconstriction. Will cause bronchodilation and relieve bronchospasm.	**IV infusion:** **Infants & Children:** 0.05-2 mcg/kg/minute **Adults:** 2-20 mcg/kg/min	**CNS:** Nervousness, weakness, insomnia, dizziness, headache, anxiety **CV:** Palpitations, tachycardia, chest pain, hypotension following a slight rise in B/P, irregular pulse **GI:** Nausea, vomiting, ulcerations, teeth damage from sublingual tablets, dry mouth, parotid edema **Skin:** Pale, cold skin; increased sweating	**Drugs:** Decreased effects with propranolol and other beta - adrenergic blockers; dysrhythmias with general anesthesia; potentiates cardiac effects of epinephrine; possible cardiotoxic effects with theophylline **Foods:** None	* Assess baseline vital signs, ECG, blood gases, CVP, and urine output. * Provide meticulous oral care to avoid mucosal and tooth damage from sublingual administration. * Compatible with most IV solutions. * Most stable in alkaline solutions. * Patient/parent education: - Teach correct administration technique. - Do not exceed recommended dose. - Contact MD if side effects occur. - Perform meticulous oral care. - Notify MD if rebound broncho- spasms occur. * IV push not established in pediatric patients; max concentration: 100 mcg/mL. * Continuous monitoring of ECG and prompt attention to chest pain or ischemic ECG changes are manda- tory.
Generic: Lidocaine **Trade:** Zylocaine	Antiarrhythmic that depresses myocardial activity and is used to treat ventricular dysrhythmias.	**IV:** Antiarrhythmic: 0.5-1.0 mg/kg/bolus repeated prn q 5-10 minutes. Maintenance infusion of 10-50 mcg/kg/ min may be utilized, pm and should not exceed 4 mg/min	**CNS:** Drowsiness, confusion, dizziness, impaired vision, paresthesia, tremors, seizures, coma **CV:** Bradycardia, hypotension **Resp:** Respiratory arrest **GI:** Nausea, vomiting **Sensory:** Tinnitus, visual disturbances **Other:** Hypersensitivity reaction	**Drugs:** Increased cardiac depressant effects with phenytoin, propranolol, other antiarrhythmics; increased hepatic metabolism with phenytoin, decreased effects with barbiturates, increased neuromuscular blocking with succinylcholine; decreased hepatic clearance and toxicity with cimetidine and propranolol. **Foods:** None	* Monitor baseline vital signs. * Have resuscitation equipment readily available. * Do not mix with other medications and solutions. * Monitor for CNS and CV side effects. * Constantly monitor ECG and B/P with IV infusion. * Monitor serum electrolytes. * Monitor serum lidocaine levels.

Table 8. DIURETICS

Name	Uses	Route and Dose	Adverse Reactions/ Side Effects	Drug or Food Interactions	Nursing Considerations
Generic: Chlorothiazide Trade: Diuril	Short-acting, potassium sparing diuretic used to treat hypertension and with digitalis to treat congestive heart failure.	PO: < 6 mo: 10-40 mg/kg/day in 1-2 doses > 6 mo & children: 10-20 mg/kg/day in 1-2 doses	CNS: Fatigue, headache, weakness, mood changes CV: Orthostatic hypotension, irregular pulse GI: Nausea, vomiting, anorexia, abdominal cramping, dry mouth, thirst Hepatic: Hepatic dysfunction Metabolic: Hypokalemia, hyponatremia, hypochloremic alkalosis, hyperuricemia, hypercalcemia, hypophosphatemia, hyperglycemia, glycosuria in diabetic patients Hemic: Thrombocytopenia, eosinophilia Other: Hypersensitivity reaction	Drugs: Increased susceptibility to digitalis toxicity and blocking effects of neuromuscular blocking agents due to hypokalemia; added risk of hypokalemia when administered with other drugs having the same effect; possible hyperglycemia with diabetic patients; added effects with other drugs causing orthostatic hypotension. Foods: None	* Assess baseline vital signs, CBC, serum electrolytes and glucose, uric acid, weight prior to administration. * Administer po form in early am and prior to meals. * Monitor hydration status. * Monitor blood glucose carefully in diabetic patients. * Monitor for signs of hypokalemia. * Patient/parent education: - Take early in the day and at the same time each day. - May take with food. - Eat potassium rich foods while taking this drug. - Get up slowly to avert orthostatic hypotension. - Avoid added sodium. - Avoid OTC medications that may contain sodium. - Monitor weight and report changes to MD. - Avoid exposure to sun. - Monitor for nausea, vomiting, and diarrhea and report to MD. - If diabetic, monitor blood glucose carefully.

Name	Uses	Route and Dose	Adverse Reactions/ Side Effects	Drug or Food Interactions	Nursing Considerations

Generic: Furosemide
 	
Trade: Lasix
	Rapid acting loop diuretic that works to inhibit sodium reabsorption at the Loop of Henle. Increases potassium excretion in distal tubules. Used to treat edema that accompanies renal failure, congestive heart failure, cerebral edema, pulmonary edema, congenital heart disease, and nephrotic syndrome.	Premature neonates: IM, IV: 1-2 mg/kg/dose given every 12-24 hrs
		
		Oral: Bioavailability is poor by this route; doses of 1q-4 mg/kg/dose 1-2 times per day have been used.
		
		Children: IM, IV: Initial 1 mg/kg/dose, increasing by 1 mg/kg/dose with each dose at intervals of 6-12 hrs; maximum 6 mg/kg/dose; continuous infusion: 0.05-0.1 mg/kg/ hour
		
		Oral: Initial: 1-8 mg/kg/day divided every 6-12 hrs.
			CNS: Vertigo, tinnitus, headache, confusion, fatigue
			CV: Orthostatic hypotension, irregular or weak pulse
			GI: Nausea, vomiting, dry mouth, thirst, stomach pain, diarrhea, anorexia
			Hepatic: Jaundice, hepatic dysfunction
			GU: Profound diuresis
			Metabolic: hypokalemia, hyponatremia, hypochloremic alkalosis
			Sensory: Tinnitus, deafness, vision changes, photosensitivity
			Hemic: Thrombocytopenia, neutropenia, anemia, leukopenia, aplastic anemia, agranulocytosis
				Drugs: Increased risk of ototoxicity if used with other drugs having the same risk; increased diuretic effects with indomethacin; increased risk of digitalis toxicity; potentiated effects with other diuretics; prolongs action of neuromuscular blockading agents; decreased lithium clearance; inhibits anticoagulants.
				
				Foods: None
					* Assess baseline vital signs, hydration status, and serum electrolytes.
					* Weigh patient.
					* Give po forms in the am to prevent nocturia and with food to decrease gastric upset.
					* Do not mix IV preparation with acidic solutions.
					* Do not give IV faster than 4 mg/min to avoid risk of hearing loss.
					* Daily weights.
					* Monitor B/P regularly.
					* Monitor I&O.
					* Monitor diabetic patients closely for hyperglycemia.
					* Patient/parent education:
					  - Take at the same time each day and no later than 3 p.m. to avoid nocturia.
					  - Take with food.
					  - Avoid hot tubs, strenuous exercise hot weather, and alcohol.
					  - Avoid rapid position changes to avert postural hypotension.
					  - Teach patient to recognize and report signs of electrolyte imbalance.
					  - Notify MD of GI symptoms.
					  - Eat potassium-rich foods.

Name	Uses	Route and Dose	Side Effects	Interactions	Considerations
Generic: Mannitol **Trade:** Osmitrol	Osmotic diuretic that works by increasing plasma osmolality, thus increasing water loss from tissues. Also facilitates water loss and toxin excretion from kidneys. Used to reduce edema in acute renal failure, cerebral and pulmonary edema, to decrease intra-ocular pressure, and to facilitate excretion of toxic substances resulting from overdose.	Children & Adults: Initial: 0.5-1.0 g/kg Maintenance: 0.25-0.5 g/kg every 4-6 hrs Intracranial pressure: IV: 0.25 g/kg/dose every 3-5 mins; may repeat at 5-min intervals as needed. Preoperative for neurosurgery: 1.5-2 g/kg/dose infused over 30-60 mins	**CNS:** Confusion, paresthesia, weakness, headache, dizziness, blurred vision, seizures **CV:** Chest pain, tachycardia **Resp:** Dyspnea, wheezing, coughing **GI:** Nausea, vomiting, thirst **GU:** Increased urination, urinary retention, renal failure following large doses **Skin:** Rash, hives, edema and/or necrosis with extravasation **Metabolic:** Hypovolemia, hyponatremia, hyperkalemia	**Drugs:** Potentiates other diuretics; hypokalemia may increase risk of digitalis toxicity; increases lithium excretion. **Food:** None	* Monitor baseline vital signs and serum electrolytes. * Weigh patient daily. * Assess hydration status. * Monitor vital signs and serum electrolytes frequently. * I&O. * Monitor for signs of hypovolemia and electrolyte imbalances. * Avoid extravasation. * Monitor for signs of rebound increased intracranial or intraocular pressure, which may occur approximately 12h following cessation of therapy.
Generic: Spironolactone **Trade:** Aldactone	Potassium sparing diuretic, often in combination with chlorothiazide.	**PO:** Hypertension/edema: 3.3 mg/kg/day in 1-4 doses; may be adjusted upward pm after 5 days of therapy	**CNS:** Lethargy, confusion, fatigue, dizziness, headache **CV:** Dysrhythmias **GI:** Nausea, vomiting, anorexia, abdominal cramping, diarrhea, dry mouth, thirst **Hepatic:** Elevated BUN **GU:** Menstrual abnormalities, breast enlargement **Metabolic:** Hyperkalemia, metabolic acidosis, hyponatremia **Skin:** Rash, urticaria, sweating	**Drugs:** Hypoglycemia in patients on insulin; hyperkalemia with potassium supplements, captopril; reduced excretion of digoxin; inhibited inotropic effects of digitalis; decreased effects with salicylates; potassium excretion potentiated with corticosteroids; potentiated by other diuretics; reduced clearance of lithium; potentiated by other potassium sparing drugs **Foods:** None	* Assess and monitor baseline vital signs, CBC, BUN, creatinine, ECG, serum electrolytes, and weight. * Tablets may be compounded into a suspension. * Refrigerate suspension and discard after 1 month. * Give with food. * Monitor for signs of hyperkalemia. * Monitor blood glucose in diabetic patients. * Patient/parent education: - Avoid potassium rich foods. - Teach signs of hyperkalemia. - Report any adverse effects to MD.

Table 9. GASTROINTESTINAL MEDICATIONS

Name	Uses	Route and Dose	Adverse Reactions/ Side Effects	Drug or Food Interactions	Nursing Considerations
Generic: Aluminum Hydroxide **Trade:** Mylanta	Antacid that neutralizes gastric acid. Used to treat gastritis and peptic ulcers.	**PO:** Ulcer: 5-15 ml/dose q 3-6h or 1-3h following meals and HS Prophylaxis against GI Bleeding: infants: 2-5 ml/dose q 1-2h children: 5-15 ml/dose q 1-2h	**GI:** Constipation, anorexia, intestinal obstruction, fecal impaction **Other:** Hypophosphatemia, hypercalciuria, dementia resulting from aluminum toxicity	**Drugs:** Interferes with absorption of tetracyclines, digoxin, phenytoin, isoniazid, iron, chlorpromazine, and ranitidine. **Foods:** None	* Shake suspension well prior to administering and follow dose with a small amount of water or milk. * Chew tablets well to ensure maximum absorption. * If given per feeding tube, validate tube placement and patency prior to administering and flush with water following dose. * Monitor for constipation. * Maintain fluid intake for age. * Patient/parent education: - Take only in amount and frequency scheduled. - Monitor for constipation. - Maintain fluid intake. - Avoid OTC drugs with MD permission.
Generic: Cimetidine **Trade:** Tagamet	Antihistamine that reduces acid secretion in the stomach by interfering with HCl receptor sites. Used to treat GI hemorrhage, peptic ulcer, hypersecretory syndrome, GE reflux, and as adjunct with severe pancreatic insufficiency that fails to respond to oral pancreatic enzyme supplements.	**PO:** 20-40 mg/kg/day q 6h, following meals and HS **IM,IV:** 20-40 mg/kg/day q 6h. Max dose = 2400 mg/day	**CNS:** Dizziness, headache, agitation, restlessness, confusion, depression, delirium, hallucinations **CV:** Bradycardia, hypotension **GI:** Mild, transient diarrhea **Hepatic:** Increase in SGOT, SGPT, alkaline phosphatase **GU:** Transient rise in serum creatinine, BUN **Hemic:** Neutropenia, agranulocytosis, thrombocytopenia, aplastic anemia **Endocrine:** Mild gynecomastia following 1 month of treatment **Other:** Muscular pain	**Drugs:** Decreased action if given with antacids; potentiates warfarin; reduces hepatic metabolism of phenytoin, lidocaine, and theophylline; decreased effectiveness with smoking **Foods:** None	* Assess stool quantity and quality with cystic fibrosis patients. * Assess PT if on warfarin therapy. * Usually given 1 hour prior to meals. * Do not give with antacids. * Do not administer IM or IV if precipitate or discoloration of preparation noted. * IM injection painful. * Must dilute prior to IV administration. * Infuse over at least 2 minutes. * Monitor for side effects. * Patient/parent education: - Follow prescribed regime. - Avoid sudden stoppage of drug to avoid ulcer perforation. - Notify MD of side effects. - Continue follow-up with MD. - Do not take OTC drugs with MD permission.

Name	Uses	Route and Dose	Adverse Reactions/ Side Effects	Drug or Food Interactions	Nursing Considerations

Generic: Glycopyrrolate
 	
Trade: Robinul
	Synthetic anticholinergic used to inhibit GI and GU motility and decrease volume of gastric and pancreatic secretions. Used in management of peptic ulcer and other GI diseases associated with hyperacidity, hypermotility, and spasm.	PO:
		> 12 yr: 1 mg TID. Max dose = 8 mg/day
		
		IM, IV:
		0.1-0.2 mg as a single dose
			CNS: Drowsiness, weakness, dizziness
			CV: Palpitation, tachycardia
			GI: Constipation
			GU: Urinary hesitancy or retention
			Sensory: Blurred vision
			Other: Decreased sweating
				Drugs: Incompatible with chloramphenicol, diazepam, sodium pentobarbital, sodium bicarbonate, or other drugs that may raise pH > 6.
				
				Food: None
					* Monitor vital signs.
					* Monitor I&O.
					* Patient/parent education:
					  - Avoid high environmental temperature.
					  - Avoid operating heavy machinery.
					  - Take only as directed.
					  - Report adverse side effects to MD.

Generic: Metoclopromide Hydrochloride
 	
Trade: Reglan
	Antiemetic used to treat GE reflux.	Gastroesophageal reflux: Infants & children: Oral: 0.1 mg/kg/dose up to 4 times/day; total daily dose should not exceed 0.5 mg/kg.
		
		Gastrointestinal hypomotility: Oral: IM, IV: Infants & children: 0.1 mg/kg/dose up to 4 times/day, the total daily dose should not exceed 0.5 mg/kg.
			CNS: Restlessness, lassitude, drowsiness, fatigue, insomnia, dizziness, headache, extrapyramidal symptoms
			CV: Transient hypertension
			GI: Constipation, diarrhea, dry mouth
			Skin: Maculopapular rash, urticaria, glossal or periorbital edema
				Drugs: Potentiates depressive effects of opiates, analgesics, anticolinergics, sedatives, alcohol, barbiturates, and tranquilizers; decreased absorption of digoxin; increased absorption of acetaminophen, salicylates, diazepam, ethanol, levodopa, lithium, and tetracycline; increased incidence of extrapyramidal side effects with phenothiazines and butyrophenones.
				
				Foods: None
					* Assess and monitor baseline vital signs.
					* Give 30 minutes prior to meals and HS for GE reflux.
					* Give slow IV push over at least 2 minutes.
					* Protect intermittent IV infusion bags from light.
					* Consult pharmacist prior to mixing with any other drug.
					* Monitor for extrapyramidal reactions 24 to 48 hours after administration.
					* Treat extrapyramidal reactions with diaphenhydramine.
					* Patient/parent education:
					  - Teach side effects.
					  - Teach proper administration.

Name	Uses	Route and Dose	Adverse Reactions/ Side Effects	Drug or Food Interactions	Nursing Considerations
Generic: Ranitidine Hydrochloride **Trade:** Zantac	Antihistamine that prohibits HCl secretion by binding with HCl receptor sites. Used to treat active GI hemorrhage, peptic ulcer disease, hypersecretory syndrome, and GE reflux.	Infants & children: Oral: 1.5-2.3 mg/kg/dose every 12 hrs IM, IV: 0.5-1 mg/kg/dose every 6-8 hrs Continuous infusion: 0.1-0.15 mg/kg/hr (preferred for stress ulcer prophylaxis in patients with concurrent maintenance IVs or TPNs)	**CNS:** Headache, dizziness, malaise, insomnia **CV:** Bradycardia, tachycardia **GI:** Nausea, constipation, abdominal discomfort **Hepatic:** Increase in SGOT, SGPT, alkaline phosphatase, LDH, total bilirubin, jaundice **Skin:** Maculopapular rash, urticaria, pruritus **Hemic:** Leukopenia, granulocytopenia, agranulocytosis, thrombocytopenia **Other:** Hypersensitivity reaction	**Drugs:** Decreased action with antacids; decreased absorption and increased serum levels of ranitidine with propantheline bromide; decreased effectiveness with smoking. **Foods:** None	* May give with meals. * If only given once per day, give HS for best results. * Do not use IM or IV preparation if discolored or contains precipitate. * Dilute IV to a concentration of 2 mg/ml and give slowly. * Assess for side effects. * Assess effectiveness. * Patient/parent education: - Follow prescribed dosage and administration times. - Notify MD if side effects occur. - Continue follow-up with MD. - Do not take OTC drugs without MD permission. - Adhere to prescribed diet.

Name	Uses	Route and Dose	Side Effects	Drug or Food Interactions	Nursing Considerations

Generic: Dexamethasone
 	
Trade: Decadron
	Corticosteroid used for its anti-inflammatory, immunosuppressant, and metabolic effects. Used for collagen, dermatologic, allergic, and leukemic diseases, as replacement therapy in adrenocortical deficiencies, and in inhaler form with asthma and rhinitis.	**Neonates:** BPD ventilator wean: 0.5 mg/kg/day for 3 days, then 0.3 mg/kg for 3 days, then reduce dose by 10% every 3 days until a dose of 0.1 mg/kg is reached; after 3 days at this dose, decrease dose every other day for 1 week then discontinue.
		Children:
		Anti-inflammatory: Oral, IM, IV: 0.03-0.15 mg/kg/24 hrs in divided doses every 6-12 hrs.
		Extubation: Oral, IM, IV: 2 mg/kg/24 hrs in divided doses every 6 hrs beginning 12 hrs prior to extubation.
		Airway edema: IV: 0.3-0.5 mg/kg/dose every 6 hrs.
		Cerebral edema: Loading dose: 1-2 mg/kg/dose as a single dose; maintenance: 1.5 mg/kg/24 hrs in divided doses every 4-6 hrs for 5 days, then taper over 5 days, then discontinue.
		Anti-emetic dose: IV: Initial: 10 mg/m2, followed by 5-10 mg/m2/dose every 6 hrs; maximum: 20 mg.
		Bacterial meningitis in infants and children >2 months: IV: 0.-6 mg/kg/24 hrs in 4 divided doses (every 6 hrs) for the first 4 days of antibiotic treatment; start dexamethasone at the time of the first dose of antibiotic.
			CNS: Headache, vertigo, euphoria, insomnia, increased ICP, psychotic behavior, seizures
			CV: Edema, hypertension, congestive heart failure
			GI: Nausea, vomiting, change in appetite, GI irritation, abdominal distention, pancreatitis, ulcerative esophagitis, peptic ulcer
			Skin: Impaired wound healing, fragile skin, petechia, ecchymosis, acne, facial erythema, increased sweating, burning, itching, irritation, dryness, folliculitis, hypertrichosis, hypo-pigmentation, allergic contact dermatitis, maceration, secondary infection, skin atrophy, striae, miliaria
			Hemic: Thrombocytopenia
			Endocrine: HPA-axis suppression, menstrual irregularities, Cushing's states, secondary adrenocortical insufficiency, pituitary unresponsiveness
			Musculoskeletal: Bone growth suppression, osteoporosis, muscle weakness, aseptic necrosis of femoral and humeral heads
			Sensory: Posterior subcapsular cataracts, increased intraocular pressure
			Other: Sodium retention, negative nitrogen balance, hypokalemia, hyperglycemia, increased susceptibility to infections
				Drugs: Increased risk of hepatotoxicity with high doses of acetaminophen; decreased risk of gastric ulceration with analgesics and anti-inflammatory drugs; increased risk of hypokalemia with amphotericin B and potassium-depleting diuretics; decreases effects of anticoagulants; lowered seizure threshold with anticonvulsants; may potentiate live virus vaccines.
				
				Foods: None
					* Obtain baseline weight and height.
					* Do not use ophthalmic preparation if eye is infected.
					* Do not use during acute asthma attack.
					* Take with food to decrease GI irritation.
					* Do not give IM doses in deltoid muscle.
					* May give slow IV push.
					* Incompatible with some IV solutions and drugs — check with pharmacist prior to mixing.
					* Monitor B/P during IV infusion.
					* Observe for side effects.
					* Patient/parent education:
					  - Take medication only as directed.
					  - Do not alter dosage or stop suddenly.
					  - Demonstrate administration of all forms other than po.
					  - Monitor for and report adverse effects.
					  - Check weight daily and report sudden changes to MD.
					  - Have eyes checked q 6 weeks if on long-term therapy.
					  - Do not get skin tests or vaccinations during therapy.
					  - Observe for signs of infection.
					  - Do not use OTC medications.
					  - Do not use inhaler during asthma attack.
					  - Have child carry medical identification card.

Name	Uses	Route and Dose	Adverse Reactions/ Side Effects	Drug or Food Interactions	Nursing Considerations
Generic: Hydrocortisone **Trade:** CaldeCORT, Cortef, Hydrocortone	Short-acting glucocortico-steroid used for its anti-inflammatory, immunosup-pressant, and metabolic actions. Used to treat collagen, dermatologic, and allergic disorders.	**PO:** 0.56-8 mg/kg/day divided q 6-8h **IM:** 0.16-1 mg/kg/day divided q 12-24h **IV:** 0.16-1 mg/kg/day divided q 12-24h Adrenal Insufficiency: 1-2 mg/kg per dose x 1 then 25-50 mg/day for infants and 150-250 mg/day for children in divided doses. Status asthmaticus: loading of 4-8 mg/kg maintenance: 2-4 mg/kg/ dose every 6 hrs up to 5 days before changing to oral prednisone. **Topical:** Lotion: 0.25%, 0.5%, or 1% solutions - apply sparingly q 12-24h; 2.5% apply q day. Cream: 0.1%, 0.25%, 0.5% or 1% solutions - apply thin film q 12-24h Ointment: 0.1%, 0.5%, or 1% - apply thin film q 12-24h; 0.2% or 2.5% applied q day	**CNS:** Headache, vertigo, euphoria, insomnia, <u>increased ICP, psychotic behavior, seizures</u> **CV:** Edema, <u>hypertension,</u> <u>CHF</u> **GI:** Nausea, vomiting, change in appetite, GI irritation, abdominal distension, <u>pancreatitis, ulcerative esophagitis, peptic ulcer</u> **Skin:** Impaired wound healing, thin fragile skin, petechiae, ecchymosis, acne, facial redness, increased sweating, folliculitis, hypertrichosis, hypopigmentation, allergic contact dermatitis, maceration, secondary infection, <u>skin atrophy,</u> <u>striae, miliaria</u> **Endocrine:** <u>HPA-axis</u> <u>suppression,</u> menstrual irregularities, Cushing's states, secondary <u>adrenocortical or pituitary</u> <u>unresponsiveness</u> **Musculoskeletal:** Suppressed bone growth, osteoporosis, muscle weakness, <u>aseptic necrosis</u> <u>of femoral and humeral</u> <u>heads</u> **Other:** Sodium retention, potassium loss, susceptibility to infections, <u>hyperglycemia,</u> <u>hypokalemia,</u> withdrawal	**Drugs:** Increased risk of hepatotoxicity with high doses of acetaminophen; decreased risk of gastric ulceration with analgesics and anti-inflammatory drugs; increased risk of hypokalemia with amphotericin B and potassium-depleting diuretics; decreases effects of anticoagulants; lowered seizure threshold with anticonvulsants; may potentiate live virus vaccines. **Foods:** None	* Obtain baseline weight and height. * Take with food to decrease GI irritation. * Do not give IM doses in deltoid muscle. * May give slow IV push. * Incompatible with some IV solutions and drugs — check with pharmacist prior to mixing. * Monitor B/P during IV infusion. * Observe for side effects. * Patient/parent education: - Take medication only as directed. - Do not alter dosage or stop suddenly. - Demonstrate administration of all forms other than po. - Monitor for and report adverse effects. - heck weight daily and report sudden changes to MD. - Do not get skin tests or vaccinations during therapy. - Observe for signs of infection. - Do not use OTC medications. - Have child carry medical identification card.

Name	Uses	Route and Dose	Side Effects	Interactions	Considerations
Generic: Methylprednisolone **Trade:** Solu-medrol	Intermediate-acting glucocorticoid with strong anti-inflammatory and immunosuppressant actions. Used to treat diseases of endocrine, integumentary, collagen, and immune systems.	**Children:** Anti-inflammatory and immunosuppressive: Oral, IM, IV: 0.16-1.0 mg/kg/24 hrs. Status asthmaticus: IV: Loading: 2 mg/kg as a single dose; maintenance: 0.5-1 mg/kg/dose every 4-6 hrs. Lupus nephritis: IV: 30 mg/kg every other day for 6 doses.	**CNS:** Headache, vertigo, euphoria, insomnia, increased ICP, psychotic behavior, seizures **CV:** Edema, hypertension, CHF **GI:** Nausea, vomiting, change in appetite, GI irritation, abdominal distension, pancreatitis, ulcerative esophagitis, peptic ulcer **Skin:** Impaired wound healing, thin fragile skin, petechiae, ecchymosis, acne, facial redness, increased sweating, folliculitis, hyperthrichosis, hypopigmentation, allergic contact dermatitis, maceration, secondary infection, skin atrophy, striae, miliaria **Endocrine:** HPA-axis suppression, menstrual irregularities, Cushing's states, secondary adrenocortical pituitary unresponsiveness **Musculoskeletal:** Suppressed bone growth, osteoporosis, muscle weakness, aseptic necrosis of femoral and humeral heads **Sensory:** Posterior subcapsular cataracts, increased intraocular pressure **Other:** Sodium retention, potassium loss, susceptibility to infections, hyperglycemia, hypokalemia, withdrawal	**Drugs:** Increased risk of hepatotoxicity with high doses of acetaminophen; decreased risk of gastric ulceration with analgesics and anti-inflammatory drugs; increased risk of hypokalemia with amphotericin B and potassium-depleting diuretics; decreases effects of anticoagulants; lowered seizure threshold with anticonvulsants; may potentiate live virus vaccines. **Food:** None	* Obtain baseline weight and height. * Take with food to decrease GI irritation. * Do not give IM doses in deltoid muscle. * Do not mix IM Depo-Medrol with any other medications. * Inject IM doses deep into muscle. * May have burning and pain with IM injection. Prevent leakage into dermis and SQ tissues to avert atrophy or abscess. * May give slow IV push. * Do not interchange Solu-Medrol and Solu-Cortef . * Incompatible with some IV solutions and drugs — check with pharmacist prior to mixing. * Monitor B/P during IV infusion. * Do not leave occlusive dressing over topical applications for > 16 hrs due to increase in possible side effects. * Observe for side effects. ** Patient/parent education: - Take medication only as directed. - Do not alter dosage or stop suddenly. - Demonstrate administration of all forms other than po. - Monitor for and report adverse effects. - Check weight daily and report sudden changes to MD. - Have eyes checked q 6 weeks if on long-term therapy. - Do not get skin tests or vaccinations during therapy. - Observe for signs of infection. - Do not use OTC medications. - Have child carry medical identification card.

Name	Uses	Route and Dose	Adverse Reactions/ Side Effects	Drug or Food Interactions	Nursing Considerations

Generic: Prednisone
 	
Trade: Delta Cortef, Cortalone
	Intermediate-acting glucocorticoid with strong anti-inflammatory and immuno-suppressant actions. Used to treat diseases of endocrine, integumentary, collagen, and immune systems.	**PO:** 0.14-2 mg/kg/day divided q 6 h
		
		Nephrosis: 2 mg/kg/day q 6-8 h either for 28 days or until urine is protein free x 5 days. If proteinuria persists, may use 4 mg/kg/day q other day for 28 days.
		
		Maintenance: 2 mg/kg/ dose q other day x 28 days and tapered over 4-6 weeks
		
		Asthma: Acute — 0.5-1 mg/kg/day x 3-5 days. Severe — 5-10 mg/day.
			CNS: Euphoria, insomnia, psychotic behavior
			CV: Edema, hypertension, CHF
			GI: Nausea, vomiting, change in appetite, GI irritation, pancreatitis, peptic ulcer
			Skin: Impaired wound healing, thin fragile skin, petechiae, ecchymosis, acne, facial redness, increased sweating
			Hemic: Thrombocytopenia
			Endocrine: HPA-axis suppression, menstrual irregularities, Cushing's states, secondary adrenocortical pituitary unresponsiveness
			Musculoskeletal: Suppressed bone growth, osteoporosis, muscle weakness
			Sensory: Posterior subcapsular cataracts, increased intraocular pressure
			Other: Negative nitrogen balance, sodium retention, susceptibility to infections, hyperglycemia, hypoka-lemia, withdrawal
				Drugs: Increased risk of hepatotoxicity with high doses of acetaminophen; decreased risk of gastric ulceration with analgesics and anti-inflammatory drugs; increased risk of hypokalemia with amphotericin B and potassium-depleting diuretics; decreases effects of anticoagulants; lowered seizure threshold with anticonvulsants; may potentiate live virus vaccines.
				
				Foods: None
					* Obtain baseline weight and height.
					* Obtain ECG, chest and spinal x-rays, glucose tolerance test, and an evaluation of HPA-axis function prior to beginning long-term therapy.
					* Assess response to medication.
					* Encourage good dental care.
					* Observe for side effects.
					* Patient/parent education:
					  - Take medication only as directed.
					  - Do not alter dosage or stop sud-denly.
					  - Demonstrate administration of all forms other than po.
					  - Monitor for and report adverse effects.
					  - Check weight daily and report sudden changes to MD.
					  - Have eyes checked q 6 weeks if on long-term therapy.
					  - Do not get skin tests or vaccina-tions during therapy.
					  - Observe for signs of infection.
					  - Do not use OTC medications.
					  - Have child carry medical identification card.

Table 11. OTHER MEDICATIONS

Name	Uses	Route and Dose	Adverse Reactions/ Side Effects	Drug or Food Interactions	Nursing Considerations
Generic: Diphenhydramine **Trade:** Benadryl	Antihistamine that works by blocking histamine release. Will not reverse histamine-related response. Used to treat allergic reactions, motion sickness, vertigo, pruritus, and as a sleeping aid.	**PO:** < 9.1 kg: 6.25-12.5 mg q 4-6h > 9.1 kg: 12.5-25 mg q 4-6h **PO,IM,IV:** 5 mg/kg/day divided q 6-8h (max. dose = 300 mg/day) **Topical:** > 2 yrs: apply TID - QID **OTC:** **Not recommended for children < 6 yrs** Allergy, motion sickness: 6-12 yr: 12.5 - 25 mg q 4-6h (max. dose = 300 mg/day) > 12 yr: 25-50 mg q 4-6h (max. dose = 150 mg/day) Cough suppressant: 6-12 yr: 12.5 mg q 4h (max. dose = 75 mg/day) > 12 yr: 25 mg q 4h (max. dose = 150 mg/day) Sleeping aid: > 2 yr: 50 mg 20 min. prior to bed; do not use longer than 2 weeks	**CNS:** Altered consciousness ranging from drowsiness to deep sleep, dizziness, headaches, paradoxical excitement, restlessness, insomnia, tremors, euphoria, delirium, <u>seizures</u> **CV:** Palpitations, hypertension, hypotension, <u>cardiovascular collapse</u> **GI:** Dry mouth, nausea, vomiting, diarrhea, constipation **Resp:** Thickened bronchial secretions, nasal stuffiness, wheezing **GU:** Dysuria, urinary retention **Skin:** Photosensitivity, eczema, pruritus, papular rash, contact dermatitis **Hemic:** Leukopenia, agranulocytosis, thrombocytopenia, hemolytic anemia **Sensory:** Diplopia	**Drugs:** Potentiates depressive effects of opiates, analgesics, anticholinergics, sedatives. alcohol, barbiturates, or tranquilizers; potentiated by MAO inhibitors; potentiates oral anticoagulants. **Foods:** None	* Obtain positive identification of organism prior to starting treatment with this drug. * Obtain baseline BUN, serum creatinine, liver function tests, hematologic tests, and weight. * Do not use reconstituted medication if not clear of precipitate and/or foreign matter. * Do not mix with other medications. * Infuse very slowly (usually over 6 hours). * Protect infusion from light. * Obtain full sets of vital signs (including temperature) q 30 minutes during infusion. * Monitor for cardiovascular collapse. * Assess I&O, weight, potassium, magnesium, BUN, serum creatinine, bilirubin, alkaline phosphatase, and SGOT QD until routine dose established then q week. * Obtain weekly CBC. * Monitor for signs of hypokalemia. * Patient/parent education: - Teach proper application of topical medications. - If no improvement noted in 2 weeks, contact MD. - Treatment may last several months. - May stain clothing. - Remove lotion from hands with soap and warm water. - Remove ointment from hands with cleaning fluid. - Do not apply OTC medications over infected area with consulting MD.

Name	Uses	Route and Dose	Adverse Reactions/ Side Effects	Drug or Food Interactions	Nursing Considerations
Generic: Ipecac Syrup Trade: Same	Emetic used to treat accidental poisonings.	Infants <6 mos: Not recommended. Children: 6-12 mos: 5-10 ml followed by 10-20 ml/kg of water; repeat dose one time if vomiting does not occur within 20 mins. 1-12 yrs: 15 ml followed by 10-20 ml/kg of water; repeat dose one time if vomiting does not occur within 20 mins. >12 yrs: 30 ml followed by 200-300 ml of water; repeat dose one time if vomiting does not occur within 20 mins.	CNS: Lethargy, tremors, seizures, coma CV: Tachycardia, dysrhythmias, atrial fibrillation, cardiomyopathy, cardiotoxicity GI: Bloody diarrhea, protracted vomiting Side effects are usually related to systemic absorption that occurs when vomiting does not occur. They may also accompany eating disorders which involve using the drug to induce vomiting.	Drugs: Activated charcoal will inactivate. Food: Delayed onset if given with milk. Carbonated beverages may decrease effectiveness.	* Assess substance ingested, time ingested, amount ingested, and treatment that has occurred. * Assess vital signs. * Notify poison control prior to giving syrup of ipecac. * Do not confuse syrup of ipecac with ipecac fluid-extract! Ipecac fluid-extract has 14 times the potency and may lead to death. * Measure dose carefully. * Give 120 - 240 ml of clear or carbonated fluids with this medication. * Do not give with activated charcoal. * Onset of vomiting is 20-30 mins following administration and will continue for 2-3 hours. * Patient/parent education: - If vomiting continues longer than 2-3 hours, notify MD. - Syrup of ipecac is nonprescription and widely available. - Keep out of child's reach. - Call poison control prior to inducing vomiting. - Check expiration date prior to administering. - Review accident prevention.

Name	Uses	Route and Dose	Side Effects	Interactions	Considerations
Generic: Lindane **Trade:** Kwell, Scabene	Pediculicide used to treat scabies, head lice, body lice, and crab lice.	**Topical:** **Scabies and body lice:** Apply thin layer of 1% from chin down. Be sure to apply under fingernails. Wash off in 6-8h. **Head lice:** Shampoo with 15-30 ml, leave on 4-10 minutes and rinse. May need to reapply in 7 days to remove all newly hatched nits. **Crab lice:** Apply shampoo to pubic areas and leave on 4 minutes before rinsing.	**CNS:** Headache, dizziness, clumsiness, restlessness, irritability, <u>seizures</u> **GI:** Nausea, vomiting, mucosal irritation **Skin:** Local irritation, rash, eczema **Other:** <u>Fatal aplastic anemia, hematologic disorders</u>	**Drugs:** None **Foods:** None	* Wear gloves to apply lindane. * Bathe child prior to treatment. * Apply all over skin including creases, hands, feet, and under fingernails. * Do not apply to face or near urethra. Bathe child 6-8 hours after application. * Check for reinfestation and repeat in 7 days, if necessary. * If shampooing for head lice, use regular shampoo prior to treatment. It is essential to avoid getting into eyes or mucous membranes. * Leave shampoo on for 4-10 mins. * Rinse hair with a solution of 1/2 water and 1/2 white vinegar or liquid fabric softener and comb through with a fine toothed comb to remove all nits. * May repeat treatment in 7 days. * If eyelashes are infested, treat with petroleum jelly rather than lindane. * Patient/parent education: - All bedding, clothing, and bath liners should be washed in hot water and dried for at least 20 mins on hot. - Combs and brushes should be soaked in a lindane solution. - All family members should be treated. - Upholstery should be professionally cleaned or cushions may be placed in a sealed plastic bag for 48 hrs then vacuumed well. - School, day care should be notified. - Recheck the child in 1 week for reinfestation.

Name	Uses	Route and Dose	Adverse Reactions/ Side Effects	Drug or Food Interactions	Nursing Considerations
Generic: Insulin **Trade:** Humulin L; Humulin N; Humulin R, Iletin Regular, Lente Iletin I; Lente Iletin II; NPH Iletin I; Pork NPH Iletin II; Pork Regular Iletin II; Regular Iletin I; Regular Iletin I, Regular Pork Insulin **Generic:** Isophane Insulin, Suspension **Trade:** NPH, Beef NPH, Iletin II, Humulin N, Iletin NPH **Generic:** Isophane Insulin, Suspension and Insulin Human **Trade:** Initard, Mixtard **Generic:** Isophane Insulin, Human, Suspension and Insulin Human **Trade:** Novolin 70/30 **Generic:** Insulin Zinc, Suspension **Trade:** Beef Lente, Iletin II, Humulin L, Lente Iletin I, Lente Insulin **Generic:** Extended Insulin, Zinc Suspension (Ultralente Insulin) Suspension **Trade:** Ultralente, Ultralente Iletin I, Ultralente purified Beef **Generic:** Prompt Insulin Zinc (Semilente) **Trade:** Semilente, Semilente Iletin I, Semilente purified Pork	Endogenous hormone secreted by beta cells in the pancreas that allow glucose transport into the cells.	**Individualized per child. Factors such as stress, illness, activity, and growth periods are considered when adjusting dose(s) to achieve control.	**Skin:** Uriticarial reactions resembling allergic reactions; local wheal or indurated area beginning approximately 20 minutes following injection and taking 7 days-3 months to subside; or insulin lipodystrophy (dimpling and atrophy of fatty tissue) **Endocrine:** Hypoglycemia, somogyi effect (rebound hyperglycemia), hyperglycemia **Other:** Allergic reactions	**Drugs:** Increased blood glucose levels with adrenocorticoids, glucocorticoids, amphetamines, contraceptives, corticotropin, dextrothyroxine, diuretics, epinephrine, glucagon, phenytoin, and thyroid hormone; potentiated hypoglycemic effects with anabolic steroids, androgens, disopyramide, salicylates, anti-inflammatory analgesics, alcohol, and beta-adrenergic blocking agents; insulin absorption decreased by smoking. **Foods:** Avoid concentrated sugars, saturated fats, cholesterol, and salt	* Assess for symptoms of hyper- or hypoglycemia. * Assess knowledge level and ability/willingness to manage care. * All brands except concentrated iletin II, U-500 available OTC. * Do not store U-500 with other types of insulin to avoid accidental substitution * Do not substitute types of insulin or brands of insulin or syringes to avoid inaccurate dosing. * Rotate injection sites. * Record site used in nurses' notes. * Allow alcohol to dry on injection site before injecting insulin to avoid precipitation of insulin. * Regular insulin is clear and should not have precipitate. * Regular insulin is the only form that may be given IV. * NPH insulin is cloudy in appearance. * Roll NPH to mix — do not shake to avoid air bubbles. * Always draw up clear (regular) insulin before NPH to avoid contamination of regular insulin. * Do not mix NPH with lente. * Roll lente, ultralente, and semilente to mix — do not shake. * Semilente may only be mixed with lente and ultralente. * Do not use semilente for ketoacidosis. * Monitor child for response (including Somogyi effect). * Monitor fluid balance and serum potassium during diabetic ketoacidosis (DKA). * Ensure that all meals and snacks are given on time. *(con't on next page)*

Name	Uses	Dose	Side Effects	Interactions	Considerations
					* Patient/parent education: - Assign one nurse to do education. - Approach teaching/education on correct developmental level for both child and parents. - Involve child in care. - Teach child first, if possible, and have child teach parents. - There should always be extra syringes and a spare vial of insulin for emergencies. - Signs and symptoms of hypo- or hyperglycemia. - Meal planning and preparation. - Foot care. - Dental care. - Eye examinations. - Child should wear medical alert jewelry. - School, day care, etc. should be notified and know proper response for hyper and hypoglycemia. - Stress importance of continuing medical follow up.

Column headers (partially visible): Dose (Route and Dose), Side Effects (Adverse Reactions/Side Effects), Interactions (Drug Interactions)

APPENDIX H
HOME CARE

Home Care Nursing Practice is defined as "... a unique combination of community health and acute care nursing provided in the client's home," (Lowdermilk, et al., 1997, p. 84). The practice may be general (infants to elderly) or specialized (oncologic, pediatric, prenatal, etc.). The employer may be a hospital, hospital system, independent agency, or third party payer.

Home care of pediatric clients is not a new concept. Over time the term has referred to parents caring for mildly ill children at home, to nursing home visits after children are discharged from the hospital to hospice care, and, more recently, to care at home for children with more serious chronic illness and dependence on medical technology (Wong, 1991).

ASPECTS OF CARE COORDINATION

– **ASSESS NEEDS**
  * Assess medical, nursing, and other needs of child
  * Assess resources and needs of family
  * Assess home environment
  * Assess resources of community

– **PLAN FOR COMPREHENSIVE CARE**
  * Develop overall integrated plan of care
  * Combine plans of venous disciplines
  * Highlight family goals
  * Assure health maintenance needs are addressed

– **LINK CLIENT(S) WITH SERVICE PROVIDER**
  * Provide information about available services
  * Initiate referrals to desired services
  * Arrange appointments
  * Assist with transportation arrangements

– **COORDINATE SERVICES**
  * Specify responsibilities of family and service providers
  * Obtain agreements
  * Help avoid service duplication
  * Arrange conferences as necessary
  * Assist in troubleshooting and problem solving between family and service providers

– **MONITOR AND EVALUATE PROVISION**
  * Maintain regular contact with family and provider

- * Review care plan on a regular basis.
- * Supervise quality of care
- * Assess safety in provision of care
- * Assess family satisfaction with care provided

- **ADVOCATE FOR APPROPRIATE SERVICES**
  - * Address problem areas in home care services
  - * Encourage educational opportunities
  - * Negotiate insurance coverage
  - * Lobby for needed services and benefits

- **PROVIDE ADMINISTRATIVE SUPPORT**
  - * Inventory equipment and supplies
  - * Assist in financial planning
  - * Complete paperwork for other insurance agencies
  - * Oversee scheduling of provider visits and appointments

From Ahmann, E.: An overview of issues in pediatric high tech home care. In Gorski L: *High tech home cure manual*, Gathersburg, MD, 1994, Aspen.

APPENDIX I
Resource Information

AIDS Hotline 1-800-447-AIDS

American Academy of Pediatrics
Publication Department
P.O. Box 927
141 Northwest Point Rd.
Elk Grove Village, IL 60009-0927

American Academy of Pediatrics Committee on Injury & Poison Prevention
The Injury Prevention Program (TIPP)
AAP
Department of Publications
P.O. Box 927
141 Northwest Point Rd.
Elk Grove Village, IL 60009-0927

American Burn Association
New York-Cornell Medical Center
525 E. 68th Street, Rm. F758
New York, NY 10021

American Cancer Society
1599 Clifton Road, N.E.
Atlanta, GA 30329

American Celiac Society
Dept. N83, 45 Gifford Ave.
Jersey City, NJ 07304

American Cleft Palate Education Foundation, Inc.
331 Salk Hall
University of Pittsburgh
Pittsburgh, PA 15261

American Diabetes Association, Inc.
2 Park Ave
New York , NY 10010

American Foundation for the Blind
15 West 16th Street
New York, NY 10011

American Heart Association
7271 Greenville Ave.
Dallas, TX 75231-4596

American Lung Association
P.O. Box 596-COL
New York, NY 10001

Arthritis Foundation/American Juvenile Arthritis Foundation
1314 Spring Street N.W.
Atlanta, GA 30309-2898

Association of Birth Defects in Children
5400 Diplomat Circle, Suite 270
Orlando, FL 32812

Asthma and Allergy Foundation of America
1125 - 15th Street, NW
Washington, D.C. 20005

Cancer Information Clearinghouse
National Cancer Institute
Office of Cancer Communication
Building 31, Room 10-A-16
9000 Rockville Pike
Bethesda, MD 20892

Candlelighters Childhood Cancer Foundation
7910 Woodmont Ave., Suite 460
Bethesda, MD 20814-3015

Celiac Sprue Association/American Celiac Society
58 Museno Court
West Orange, NJ 07052

Centers for Disease Control and Prevention (CDC) Injury Prevention
4770 Buford Highway
Atlanta, GA 30344

Consumer Product Safety Commission
Office of Information
Washington, DC 20207

Cystic Fibrosis Foundation
6931 Arlington Road, #200
Bethesda, MD 20814

Epilepsy Foundation of America
4351 Garden City Dr.
Landover, MD 20785

Immunization Practices Advisory Committee
U.S. Dept. of Health & Human Services
Centers for Disease Control
Atlanta, GA 30333

Juvenile Diabetes Foundation International
120 Wall Street
New York, NY 10005

Leukemia Society of America
600 Third Street, 4th Floor
New York, NY 10006

March of Dimes Birth Defects Foundation
1275 Mamaroneck Ave
White Plains, NY 10605

Muscular Dystrophy Association of America
10 East 40th Street, Room 4110
New York, NY 10016

National Arthritis & Musculoskeletal & Skin Diseases Information Clearinghouse
P.O. Box AMS
9000 Rockville Pike
Bethesda, MD 20892

National Association of the Deaf
American Society for Deaf Children
814 Thayer Avenue
Silver Spring, MD 20910-4500

National Association for Parents of the Visually Impaired, Inc.
P. O. Box 317
Watertown, MA 02272-0317

National Association of Patients on Hemodialysis and Transplantation
150 Nassau Street
New York, NY 10038

National Association for Sickle Cell Disease, Inc.
200 Corporate Pointe, Suite 495
Culver City, CA 90203-7633

National Center for Health Statistics
Dept. of Health and Human Services
Public Health Services
3700 East-West Highway
Hyattsville, MD 20782

National Center for Learning Disabilities (NCLD)
99 Park Avenue, 6th Floor
New York, NY 10016

National Child Safety Council
4065 Page Ave
P. O. Box 1368
Jackson, MI 49204

National Diabetes Information Clearinghouse
9000 Rockville Pike
P.O. Box NDIC
Bethesda, MD 20892

National Down's Syndrome Society
666 Broadway, Suite 810
New York, NY 10012-2317

National Hearing Aid Society
20361 Middlebelt Rd.
Livonia, MI 48152

National Heart, Lung and Blood Institute
National Institutes of Health
Bethesda, MD 20824-0105

National Hemophilia Foundation
110 Green Street, Room 303
New York, NY 10012

National Kidney Foundation
30 East 33rd Street, 11th Floor
New York, NY 10016

National Reye's Syndrome Foundation
P.O. Box 829
Bryon, OH 43506

National Scoliosis Foundation
72 Mount Auburn St.
Watertown, MA 02172

National Easter Seals Society
70 East Lake Street
Chicago, IL 60601

Osteogenesis Imperfecta Foundation
P.O. Box 14807
Tampa, FL 34629-4807

Parent's Anonymous
675 W. Foothill Blvd., Suite 220
Claremont, CA 91711

Spina Bifida Association of America
4590 MacArthur Blvd., NW, Suite 250
Washington, DC 20207-4226

Sudden Infant Death Syndrome Resource Center
2070 Chain Bridge Road
Vienna, VA 22182

The Compassionate Friends
P. O. Box 3696
Oak Brook, II 60522-3696

United Cerebral Palsy Association
1660 L Street, NW., Suite 700
Washington, DC 20036

United Ostomy Association
36 Executive Park, Suite 120
Irvine, CA 92714-6744

INTERNET RESOURCES

Promoting Injury Prevention
Global Childnet: http://www.gcnet.org/gcnet
PedInfo: http://www.lhl.uab.edu/pedinfo/Aboutr.html
American Academy of Pediatrics: http://www.aap.org

Information on technology improvements in health care cost, quality and access
http://www.cpri.org

Generic Pediatric Internet Resources
American Academy of Pediatrics: http://www.aap.org
Children's Defense Fund: http://www.tmn.com/cd/index.html
Global Childnet: http://www.gcnet.org/gcnet
Parents Place: http://www.parentsplace.com
PedInfo: http://lhl.uab.edu/pedinfo/miscellaneous.html
Positive Parenting On Line: http://www.fishnet.net/
Resources of Nurses, Children and Families:
        http://pegasus.cc.ucf.edu/~wink/home.html

Cardiac
American Heart Association: http://www.amhrt.org

Developmental Disabilities
Spina Bifida: Parents of children with spina bifida discussion list: bifida-1
        To subscribe, send message to: listserv@nervm.nerdc.ufl.edu
        In message type: subscribe cshcn-1 <your first name> <your last name>
        Send mail to: cshcn-1@yalevm.cis.yale.edu
Spina Bifida Hydrocephalus:
        To subscribe, send message to: listserv@mercury.dsu.edu
        Spina Bifida web page: http://www.familyvillage.wisc.edu/lib_spin.htm
Cystic Fibrosis support discussion list: cystic-1
        To subscribe, send message to: listserve@yalem.cis.yale.edu
        In message type: subscribe cystic-1 <your first name> <your last name>
        Send mail to the following: cystic-1@yalevm.cis.yale.edu

Asthma

http://www.plsgroup.com/asthma
http://www.ginasthma.com/asthma
http://www.remcomp.com/asthmanet

APPENDIX J
Abbreviations Related to Pediatrics

ADD - Attention deficit disorder

ADHD - Attention deficit hyperactivity disorder

ADL - Activity of daily living

AFP - Alpha feto protein

AGN - Acute glomerulonephritis

AIDS - Acquired immunodeficiency syndrome

ALL - Acute lymphocytic leukemia

AML - Acute myelocytic leukemia

ANLL - Acute nonlymphocytic leukemia

ARF - Acute renal failure

ASD - Atrial septal defect

BMT - Bone marrow transplant

BP - Blood pressure

BPD - Bronchopulmonary dysplasia

CF - Cystic fibrosis

CHD - Congenital heart defect

CHF - Congestive heart failure

CIC - Clean intermittent catheterization

CNS - Central nervous system

COA - Coarctation of the aorta

CP - Cerebral palsy or cleft palate

CPR - Cardiopulmonary resuscitation

CPT - Chest physiotherapy

CRF - Chronic renal failure

CSF - Cerebrospinal fluid

CT scan - Computerized axial tomography

CVA - Cerebrovascular accident

CXR - Chest x-ray

DDST - Denver developmental screening tool

DNASE - Recombinant human deoxyribonuclease

DPT - Diphtheria, pertussis, tetanus

EBV - Epstein-Barr virus

ECG - Electrocardiogram

ECMO - Extracorporeal membrane oxygenation

EMG - Electromyelogram

ESR - Erythrocyte sedimentation rate

FAS - Fetal alcohol syndrome

FB - Foreign body

FTT - Failure to thrive

GAS - Group A streptococcus

GER - Gastroesophageal reflux

HHV-6 - Human herpes virus, type 6

HIB - Hemophilus influenza, type B

HIV - Human immunodeficiency virus

HTLV-3 - Human T-cell lymphotrophic virus, type 3

HLHS - Hypoplastic left heart syndrome

I&O - Intake and output

IgM - Immune globulin M

IgE - Immune globulin E

IICP - Increased intracranial pressure

IDDM - Insulin dependent diabetes mellitus, type I

ITP - Idiopathic thrombocytopenic purpura

IVIG - Intravenous immune globulin

JRA - Juvenile rheumatoid arthritis

LTB - Laryngotracheobronchitis

MD - Muscular dystrophy

MI - Mitral insufficiency; myocardial infarction

MMR - Measles, mumps, rubella

MR - Mental retardation

MRI - Magnetic resonance imaging

MVA - Motor vehicle accident

NAT - Nonaccidental trauma

NOFTT - Nonorganic failure to thrive

NHL - Non-Hodgkin's lymphoma

NSAID - Nonsteroidal anti-inflammatory

OI - Osteogenesis imperfecta

OT - Occupational therapy

PDA - Patent ductus arteriosus

PEFR - Peak expiratory flow rate

PFT - Pulmonary function test

PICC - Peripherally inserted central catheter

PS - Pulmonary stenosis

PT - Physical therapy

RDS - Respiratory distress syndrome

RF - Rheumatic fever; renal failure

ROP - Retinopathy of prematurity

RSV - Respiratory syncytial virus

RVH - Right ventricular hypertrophy

TEF - Tracheoesophageal fistula

TGV - Transposition of the great vessels

TIG - Tetanus immune globulin

TOF - Tetralogy of Fallot
TOPV - Trivalent oral polio vaccine
UTD - Up to date
UTI - Urinary tract infection
VCUG - Voiding cystourethrogram
VP - Ventriculoperitoneal
VS - Vital signs
VSD - Ventricular septal defect
VUR - Vesicoureteral reflux
VZIG - Varicella zoster immune globulin
VZV - Varicella zoster virus

APPENDIX K
The 1996-97 List of NANDA Nursing Diagnoses

Activity Intolerance
Activity Intolerance, Risk for
Adaptive Capacity, Decreased Intracranial
Adjustment, Impaired
Airway Clearance, Ineffective
Anxiety
Aspiration, Risk for
Body Image Disturbance
Body Temperature, Risk for Altered
Breastfeeding, Effective
Breastfeeding, Ineffective
Breastfeeding, Interrupted
Breathing Pattern, Ineffective
Cardiac Output, Decreased
Caregiver Role Strain
Caregiver Role Strain, Risk for
Communication, Impaired Verbal
Community Coping, Ineffective
Community Coping, Potential for Enhanced
Confusion, Acute
Confusion, Chronic
Constipation
Constipation, Colonic
Constipation, Perceived
Coping, Defensive
Coping, Ineffective Individual
Decisional Conflict (Specify)
Denial, Ineffective
Diarrhea
Disuse Syndrome, Risk for
Diversional Activity Deficit
Dysfunctional Ventilatory Weaning Response
Dysreflexia
Energy Field, Disturbance
Environmental Interpretation Syndrome, Impaired
Family Coping, Compromised, Ineffective
Family Coping, Disabling, Ineffective
Family Coping, Potential for Growth
Family Processes, Altered
Family Processes, Altered; Alcoholism
Fatigue
Fear
Fluid Volume Deficit

Fluid Volume Deficit, Risk for
Fluid Volume Excess
Gas Exchange, Impaired
Grieving, Anticipatory
Grieving, Dysfunctional
Growth and Development, Altered
Health Maintenance, Altered
Health-Seeking Behaviors (Specify)
Home Maintenance Management, Impaired
Hopelessness
Hyperthermia
Hypothermia
Incontinence, Bowel
Incontinence, Functional
Incontinence, Reflex
Incontinence, Stress
Incontinence, Total
Incontinence, Urge
Infant Behavior, Disorganized
Infant Behavior, Potential for Enhanced Organized
Infant Behavior, Risk for Disorganized
Infant Feeding Pattern, Ineffective
Infection, Risk for
Injury, Risk for
Knowledge Deficit (Specify)
Loneliness, Risk for
Management of Therapeutic Regimen, Effective, Individual
Management of Therapeutic Regimen, Ineffective, Community
Management of Therapeutic Regimen, Ineffective, Family
Management of Therapeutic Regimen, Ineffective, Individual
Memory, Impaired
Noncompliance (Specify)
Nutrition: Less than Body Requirements, Altered
Nutrition: More than Body Requirements, Altered
Nutrition: Potential for More than Body Requirements, Altered
Oral Mucous Membrane, Altered
Pain
Pain, Chronic
Parent/Infant/Child Attachment; Risk for Altered
Parental Role Conflict
Parenting, Altered
Parenting, Risk for Altered
Perioperative Positioning; Risk for Injury
Peripheral Neurovascular Dysfunction, Risk for
Personal Identity Disturbance
Physical Mobility, Impaired
Poisoning, Risk for
Post-Trauma Response

Powerlessness
Protection, Altered
Rape-Trauma Syndrome
Rape-Trauma Syndrome: Compound Reaction
Rape-Trauma Syndrome: Silent Reaction
Relocation Stress Syndrome
Role Performance, Altered
Self-Care Deficit: Bathing/Hygiene, Dressing/Grooming, Feeding, Toileting
Self-Esteem, Chronic Low
Self-Esteem, Situational Low
Self-Esteem, Disturbance
Self-Mutilation, Risk for
Sensory/Perceptual Alterations (Specify: Visual, Auditory, Kinesthetic, Gustatory, Tactile, Olfactory)
Sexual Dysfunction
Sexual Patterns, Altered
Skin Integrity, Impaired
Skin Integrity, Risk for
Sleep Pattern Disturbance
Social Interaction, Impaired
Social Isolation
Spiritual Distress (Distress of the Human Spirit)
Spiritual Well-being; Potential for Enhanced
Suffocation, Risk for
Swallowing, Impaired
Thermoregulation, Ineffective
Thought Processes, Altered
Tissue Integrity, Impaired
Tissue Perfusion, Altered (Specify Type: Renal, Cerebral, Cardiopulmonary, Gastrointestinal, Peripheral)
Tissue Perfusion, Altered Cardiac
Trauma, Risk for
Unilateral Neglect
Urinary Elimination, Altered
Urinary Retention
Ventilation, Inability to Sustain Spontaneous
Violence, Risk for: Self-Directed or Directed at Others

APPENDIX L
References

Behrman, R.E. and Kliegman, R.M. (1994). <u>Nelson Essentials of Pediatrics</u> (2nd ed.). Philadelphia: W.B. Saunders Company.

The Children's Hospital of Denver (1996). <u>Formulary and Drug Handbook</u>. Hudson, OH: Lexi-Comp, Inc.

Committee on Infectious Diseases (1997). <u>1997 Red Book Report of the Committee on Infectious Diseases</u> (24th ed.). Elk Grove Village, IL: American Academy of Pediatrics.

Fox, Jane A. (Ed.). (1997). <u>Primary Health Care of Children</u>. St. Louis: Mosby-Year Book, Inc.

Genevive-Foley, V., Fochtman, D. & Hardin-Money, K. (1993). <u>Nursing Care of the Child With Cancer</u>. (2nd ed.). Philadelphia: W. B. Saunders.

Graef, J.W. (Ed.). (1993) <u>Manual of Pediatric Therapeutics</u> (5th ed.). Boston: Little, Brown and Company.

Nelson, Waldo E., Behrman, Richard E., Kliegman, Robert M., Arvin, Ann M. (Eds) (1996). Philadelphia: W. B. Saunders Company.

Santesteban, Alfredo (1997). <u>The Complete Guide to Pediatric Hot-Lines and Resources</u>. Bedford, TX: ABC and F Press.

Shannon, M., Wilson, B. and Stang, C. (1995). <u>Govoni and Hays: Drugs and Nursing Implications</u> (8th ed.). Norwalk: Appleton and Lange.

Whaley, L.F. and Wong, D.L. (1995). <u>Nursing Care of Infants and Children</u> (5th ed.) St. Louis: Mosby-Year Book, Inc.

Wong, D.L. (1995). <u>Whaley and Wong's Nursing Care of Infants and Children</u>. St. Louis: Mosby-Year Book, Inc.

SKIDMORE-ROTH PUBLISHING, INC.

400 Inverness Drive South, Suite 260, Englewood, CO 80112

Ph. 1-800-825-3150

title	code	isbn #	price	qty
INSTANT INSTRUCTOR SERIES				
AIDS HIV, Bradley-Springer 1995	ADIN01	1-56930-010-0	$9.95	
C.C.U., Randall 1995	CCIN01	1-56930-022-4	$9.95	
Geriatric, Jaffe 1992	GRIN01	0-944132-68-5	$9.95	
Hemodialysis, Fowlds 1994	DLIN01	1-56930-020-8	$9.95	
I.C.U., Randall 1995	ICUI01	1-56930-021-6	$9.95	
IV, Krasner & Ray 1995	IVII01	1-56930-043-7	$9.95	
Obstetric, Jaffe 1992	OBIN01	0-944132-67-7	$9.95	
Oncology, Gale 1994	ONIN01	1-56930-023-2	$9.95	
Pediatric, Keller 1992	PDIN01	0-944132-66-9	$9.95	
Psychiatric, Yard 1992	PSYI01	0-944132-69-3	$9.95	
NURSING CARE PLANS SERIES				
Critical Care, Comer 1998	CNCP01	1-56930-035-6	$38.95	
Geriatric (2nd ed.), Jaffe 1996	GNCP02	1-56930-052-6	$38.95	
HIV/AIDS (2nd ed.), Bradley-Springer 1998	ADSC02	1-56930-097-6	$38.95	
Oncology, Gale 1996	ONCP01	1-56930-004-6	$38.95	
Pediatric (2nd ed.), Jaffe 1998	PNCP02	1-56930-057-7	$38.95	
SURVIVAL SERIES				
Geriatric Survival Handbook, Acello 1997	GSGD01	1-56930-061-5	$29.95	
Nurse's Survival Handbook, Acello 1998	NSHB01	1-56930-040-2	$39.95	
Obstetric Survival Handbook, Masten 1998	OBHB01	1-56930-083-6	$35.95	
Pediatric Nurse's Survival Guide, Rebeschi 1996	PSGD01	1-56930-018-6	$29.95	
NURSING/OTHER				
Body in Brief (3rd ed.), Rayman 1997	BBRF03	1-56930-055-0	$35.95	
Diagnostic and Lab Cards (3rd ed.), Skidmore-Roth 1998	DLC03	1-56930-065-8	$29.95	
Drug Comparison Handbook (2nd ed.), Reilly 1995	DRUG02	1-56930-16-X	$35.95	
Essential Laboratory Mathematics, Johnson & Timmons 1997	ELM01	1-56930-056-9	$29.95	
Geriatric Long-Term Procedures & Treatments (2nd ed.), Jaffe 1994	GLTP02	1-56930-072-0	$36.95	

title	code	isbn #	price	qty
Geriatric Nutrition and Diet Therapy (3rd ed.), Jaffe 1998	NUT03	1-56930-096-8	$25.95	
Handbook for Nurse Assistants (2nd ed), Nurse Asst. Consort. 1997	HNA02	1-56930-059-3	$23.95	
I.C.U. Quick Reference (2nd ed.), Comer 1998	ICQU02	1-56930-071-2	$35.95	
Infection Control, Palmer 1996	INFC01	1-56930-051-8	$99.95	
Long-Term Care: A Skills Handbook for Nurse Assistants (2nd ed.), Vitale 1998	HLTC02	1-56930-058-5	$23.95	
Nursing Diagnosis Cards (2nd ed.), Weber 1997	NDC02	1-56930-060-7	$29.95	
Nurse's Trivia Calendar, Rayman	NTC98	1-56930-073-9	$11.95	
OBRA (3rd ed.), Jaffe 1998	OBRA03	1-56930-047-X	$119.95	
OSHA Book (2nd ed.), Goodner 1997	OSHA02	1-56930-069-0	$119.95	
Pharmacy Tech, Reilly 1994	PHAR01	1-56930-005-4	$25.95	
Procedure Cards (3rd ed.), Jaffe 1996	PCCU03	1-56930-054-2	$24.95	
Spanish for Medical Personnel, Meizel 1993	SPAN01	1-56930-001-1	$21.95	
OUTLINE SERIES				
Critical and High Acuity Outline, Reynolds 1995	HATO01	1-56930-028-3	$23.95	
Fundamentals of Nursing Outline, Chin 1995	FUND01	1-56930-029-1	$23.95	
Geriatric Outline, Morice 1995	GER01	0-944132-90-1	$23.95	
Hemodynamic Monitoring Outline, Schactman 1995	HDMO01	1-56930-034-8	$23.95	
Med-Surgical Nursing Outline (2nd ed.), Reynolds 1998	MSN02	1-56930-068-2	$23.95	
Obstetric Nursing Outline (2nd ed.), Masten 1997	OBS02	1-56930-070-4	$23.95	
Pediatric Nursing Outline (2nd ed.), Froese-Fretz et al 1998	PN02	1-56930-067-4	$23.95	
RN NCLEX REVIEW SERIES				
PN/VN NCLEX Review Cards (3rd ed.), Goodner 1998	PNRC03	1-56930-093-3	$32.95	
RN NCLEX Review Cards (3rd ed.), Goodner 1998	RNRC03	1-56930-092-5	$32.95	

Name_____

Address_____

City_____ State_____ Zip_____

Phone (_____)_____

❑ VISA   ❑ MasterCard   ❑ American Express   ❑ Check/Money Order

Card #_____ Exp. Date_____

Signature (required)_____

Prices subject to change. Please add $6.95 each for postage and handling. Include your local sales tax.

MAIL ORDER TO:
    SKIDMORE-ROTH PUBLISHING, INC.
    400 Inverness Drive South, Suite 260
    Englewood, Colorado 80112
    1-800-825-3150

       Visit our website at: http://www.skidmore-roth.com